Through the Eye of the Storm

My Journey

Isa. 49:15b-16 KJV
"Yet will I not forget thee. Behold, I have graven thee upon the palms of my hands."

Donna Criswell Owens

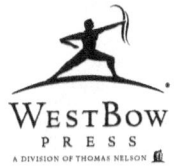

WestBow
PRESS
A DIVISION OF THOMAS NELSON

Scripture taken from the King James Version of the Bible.

Scripture taken from the New King James Version. Copyright 1979, 1980, 1982 by Thomas Nelson, inc. Used by permission. All rights reserved.

Scripture quotations are from The Holy Bible, English Standard Version® (ESV®), copyright © 2001 by Crossway, a publishing ministry of Good News Publishers. Used by permission. All rights reserved.

WestBow Press books may be ordered through booksellers or by contacting:

WestBow Press
A Division of Thomas Nelson
1663 Liberty Drive
Bloomington, IN 47403
www.westbowpress.com
1 (866) 928-1240

Because of the dynamic nature of the Internet, any web addresses or links contained in this book may have changed since publication and may no longer be valid. The views expressed in this work are solely those of the author and do not necessarily reflect the views of the publisher, and the publisher hereby disclaims any responsibility for them.

Any people depicted in stock imagery provided by Thinkstock are models, and such images are being used for illustrative purposes only.
Certain stock imagery © Thinkstock.

ISBN: 978-1-4908-1786-6 (sc)
ISBN: 978-1-4908-1787-3 (e)

Library of Congress Control Number: 2013921407

Printed in the United States of America.

WestBow Press rev. date: 11/26/2013

This book is dedicated to my husband, Michael, my sons, my daughters-in-law and my grandchildren. You are my inspiration.

Contents

Preface

With life we are given a special gift of memory. Memories are a treasure and remember that today's experiences are making tomorrow's memories. Memories can change form slightly from childhood to adult. Not all memories I have as a child may have actually been as large as they appear on these pages. Memories help us recall the journey and perhaps see some lessons the journey has taught. God has been and continues to be good to me. I am blessed with great family and friends and many loving memories. Not all who crossed my path on this journey will be named, but all who did have had an impact on my life; some known and some unknown. Some of the names may have been changed. Some joined for the entire trip and others in and out along the way. For all of you, I am thankful.

Life is full of adventure, sorrow, everyday living, excitement and the mundane. Lessons are always to be learned and the wisdom to confront every day only comes from God. This is my history, my life, my inheritance, my legacy that I pass on to my family. Gratitude for it all, good along with the bad, is what I want to convey through my journey. From my childhood, marriage, children, grandchildren, war, cancer, and transplant, this is from my perspective encircling many along the way.

Typically a journey begins with a conscious plan. An idea, an itinerary, and a couple of bags packed with anticipated needs necessary to fulfill the journey. Not so with my journey, as it begins with personal accounts from others and some court records that would verify its beginning as I fail to remember the start of this journey, and most of this journey is unplanned on my part. My desire is that you see the thread of God's hand through my journey.

Psalm 121 NKJV

"I will lift up my eyes to the hills, from whence comes my help? My help comes from the Lord who made heaven and earth. He will not allow your foot to be moved; He who keeps you will not slumber. Behold, He who keeps Israel shall neither slumber nor sleep. The Lord is your keeper. The Lord is your shade at your right hand. The sun will not strike you by the day, nor the moon by night. The Lord shall preserve you from all evil; He shall preserve your soul. The Lord shall preserve your going out and your coming in from this time forth even forevermore."

Acknowledgements

My parents receive the first acknowledgement for bringing me into this world and for all their influences that pointed me in the right direction to become the person I am today. From their perspective, I hope that I have made them proud more often than disappointed.

A special thanks to those who endured the rough copies, gave their criticism, and helped with the editing, especially my sister-in-law, Charlotte. A big thanks to my husband, Michael, who helped me fulfill this dream and for his organizational skills over the years that allowed me to keep all the dates in order.

Thanks, also, to my sons, daughters-in-law and grandchildren. All of you kept me going through the journey and provided much of my writing material.

Thanks to my family, friends, and acquaintances along the way that have participated in my life and gave direction whether they realized this or not.

The Introduction

The storm began off the coast of western Africa and barely anyone noticed. It slowly churned its way across the Atlantic until one day, as a completely organized storm, it appears on radar and the preparations begin. The preparations for this event were small. The majority of the East coast and certainly not the rest of the world would scarcely notice as this small, yet familiar action makes its way north.

Imagine those twists and churns as those in the eye of the action are only slightly aware of greater action on the edges of the storm. No one expected its beginning, and no one could predict its path or its end. Over the course of the storms' history many are affected. Some are only slightly nudged and for a short amount of time. Others are carried the length of the churning, and still some are affected as recent newcomers. All are connected by the beginning, the birth of an event. Storms have beauty, excitement and a drawing, yet can stir fear and wonder as they create adventure and intrigue. They have a beginning and an end. Yet the eye of the storm remains calm even as its energy spreads, and the circles grow.

This is life. No matter how insignificant the life, it has an impact on those surrounding it. Stepping out of the eye is chaos, but in the eye is relative peace. A greater power, a hand, a guide has it all under control. There is a plan even in the dark times as well as the bright ones, and that plan will come to fruition. Now we follow this small blip on the radar of life… through the eye of the storm.

Chapter 1

Journey Begins

According to my birth certificate I was born into the Criswell family on December 16, 1952 as Donna Lee Criswell. The name, Donna, means "Lady" but as you will see that no matter how hard Mom tried, I was a tomboy. God had me on His mind long before that day and made me according to His specifications. Psalm 139 comes to mind as we are all "fearfully and wonderfully made". My parents were only eighteen years old when I arrived. Even in those days there would have been other options. I am certainly thankful for the chance to give this life a whirl! As I entered kicking and screaming, so I would like to depart in equal manner, but of such things we have no control.

Even though I cannot seem to remember much of those early days, I have been told many stories. We were living on the third floor of Pop Pop and Nee Nee Criswell's farm house. Supposedly my dear Daddy said upon my birth, "It's a dumb ole girl!" I guess that statement has something to do with my becoming a tomboy, just to prove that girls were not DUMB! I was also the FIRST grandchild on both sides of the family. From my present vantage point as a grandmother, I now realize I had it made!

I was born in Havre de Grace, Maryland and delivered by Dr. Neil Taylor of Rising Sun, Maryland. My Mom remembers seeing the holly tree at Jackson Station on the way to the hospital, and now it always reminds me of my birth day. I guess it took her mind off the pain and my impending birth for a few minutes, and I have wondered how she could focus on a tree. Ready or not world here I come!

One of those early stories include a terrible thunder storm in which I had been left sleeping on the third floor while everyone else huddled on the first floor. My Dad's cousin's (Janice) husband, Ellis Leatherwood, came to the third floor to make sure I was okay and still sleeping. It is nice to know someone cared. Remember, I was the first grandchild on both sides of the family, and I was spoiled.

By the time I was two, Mom said I suddenly had an imaginary friend named Debbie. Debbie did everything with me. She listened and obeyed me, we sat a place at the table for her, she slept in my room, and she hung around until my sister, Lynn, was born. Then she disappeared as quickly as she came. I only regret she did not stay around long enough to teach my new sister some of those good habits, such as listening and being obedient to me! Lynn soon became my playmate and friend most of the time. Cultivating a friendship with your siblings is wise. Siblings are the best friends you can ever have. Siblings know you well and, typically, forgive easily. It is too bad we do not realize this when we are kids. Lynn was born when I was three years old, and we have had our moments, but I would defend her against anyone who tried to hurt her. Siblings often have a love/hate relationship, share secrets, and know details that no other person knows.

My Dad said I would often sit on the couch or chair and tap my foot to a song or beat that only I heard. During this time frame, I was entered in a beauty contest and won. Perhaps it was with the help of the cute dog named Good Boy that I pushed in a baby carriage. Life was good.

Mom taught me many fun things such as nursery rhymes, verses and songs and even how to jitterbug. I can sing many of those songs until this day and have taught them to my children. One little song that is still special, which I now sing to my grandchildren now and, hopefully, many other grandchildren in the future, is the following:

"I love you a bushel and a peck
A bushel and a peck and a hug around the neck
A hug around the neck and a barrel and a heap
A barrel and a heap and I'm talking in my sleep about YOU!"
(Taken from Guys and Dolls)

This song is always followed by "You are my
favorite Aiden in the whole wide world"
OR
"You are my favorite Eli in the whole wide world"
OR
"You are my favorite Liza in the whole wide world"

Every child loves to be talked, sang, and read to as often as possible. Never pass up the opportunity to read a good book, teach a new song, or tell a good story to a child. It is valuable time for you both. Story time is always snuggle time. I loved curling up on Mom's lap for a book. I always enjoyed reading books to our boys and, now, to the grandchildren. Multiple Golden Books and countless other books have become favorites over the years to our sons and, in recent years, grandchildren. These books still line our book shelf. Michael, too, spent many evening hours reading to our sons. Books can take you to a wonderful world. As they grew older, Michael read C.S. Lewis' Chronicles of Narnia to the boys. They were enjoyed as children for their wonderful stories and, although the symbolism was often too deep, they quickly picked up on Aslan and who he was in the story. Find a good book and read to a child in your life as it is not time wasted.

The Criswell farm included about 157 acres, so it kept everyone very busy milking cows, planting and harvesting crops and the countless other chores that filled each day. I remember very little of actually living on the farm, but recall many memories of farm days. Things like visiting my Great Nana who lived on the first floor in a little apartment come to mind. I loved to eat bananas and her homemade ginger cookies with her. My fond memories of my Nana are why when my grandchildren came along I wanted to be called Nana. Plus, Nana is so easy to say that they learn to speak it quickly. Most of my memories are from later years, as we visited the farm often. Dad had decided that farming was not for him, as he was a mechanic, and he started working at the Zion Garage. We left the farm and moved to several different houses; the one in Rising Sun, Maryland on Main Street is where I remember the biggest snowstorm ever. It was higher than I, at three feet deep, and Daddy threw me in a snow drift. Later we moved to an apartment on Cedar Farm where memories of Mom and Dad's friends; Claude and Jane, Frank and Ruth and Peggy and Earl are all connected in my memory. Earl brought home a silk outfit for me from Japan as he was returning from the Korean War, and I have stayed close to Peggy and Earl over the years. Remember, my parents were just kids themselves and they spent much time with their friends. Their friends were important to them and those high school friends were always there. We later moved to a house Dad and Mom bought in Zion, the perfect little village. Driving or riding my bike past the farm on England Creamy Road today still makes me smile because the memories are sweet. My injuries, as I recall, were few. Bumps and bruises are just a part of childhood. The most major injury as a little girl on the farm was cutting my right thumb on the grinder used to sharpen knives. Not a bad record for farm living. I loved riding the tractor with Pop Pop, and he taught me the shocking truth of an electric fence. Pop Pop was a happy man and liked to sing. He would often sing this song to me.

"Did you ever go afishin' on a hot summer day,
and sit on the bank just passin' time away,
with your hands in your pockets and your pockets in your pants,
and watch the little fishes do the hoochie coochie dance?"
(Author unknown)

Pop Pop always kept that bald head under a cap, wore a smile, and walked with a distinct bend from the years of hard work.

Farming was such hard work requiring 24/7 commitment, yet it was just the way life was. The milking twice a day, plowing, planting and harvesting plus all the maintenance chores and feedings made for hard, but rewarding work for my Pop Pop and the family. The garden was sizeable and required much work to keep the weeds from overtaking the plants. We ate well all year as a result of the garden with the canning and freezing of the harvest. Chicken killing day was another event to remember. Chopping off their heads, dipping them in boiling water, plucking their feathers, cleaning out the guts, and then preparing them for the freezer usually took an entire day. The few, who ran around after their heads were chopped off, made the day extra exciting. It seemed to me that they ran quite far sometimes without a head! Newborn calves, bailing hay and hundreds of farm kittens were included in farm living. The farm was a part of my life until my grandfather retired and sold it when I was a teenager.

My Mom was born Thelma Lee Clark on September 15, 1934. She is one of five children born to Fred and Mary Clark. Pop Pop Clark helped to build the Conowingo Dam on the Susquehanna River in Conowingo, Maryland. He was a proud man from Baltimore who met Mary Elizabeth Crothers while living in Conowingo as he worked on the dam. Construction of the dam was very hard work as you can imagine. Fred married Mary after ordering a diamond from Cracker Jacks. It is a real diamond and Mom Mom later gave it to my Mom. Pop Pop caused some rough days for Mom and her family over the years. God did change his heart a few years before he died and my sons remember him quite differently. He still could be gruff, such as when he yelled, "shut the door", but now he did it with a smile. During Mom's childhood, Mom Mom and the children found their way to church through CM Jones, Pastor Walter Burcham and a church in Conowingo. Mom Mom was quite a lady and hard worker. Actually, she was a happy lady and enjoyed teasing, causing mayhem, and just having fun enjoying life with her family and many friends until her death in 2001. Everyone loved Mary Clark. She was a true people person who loved taking care of others as she demonstrated throughout her life. Later in life when others are considering retirement, Mom Mom got her driver's license and worked at Calvert Manor Nursing Home. She enjoyed taking care of the "old people" as she would say.

Dad, Harold Donald Criswell, known as Donnie, Don, or Harold, if you are trying to visit him in the hospital in this decade, was born to Harold and Mildred (Sartin) Criswell on September 29, 1934. He was a tiny thing, born under 4 lbs, but his Mom nursed him and he grew much to everyone's surprise. Even the doctor told his Mom he would never make it. He is the older of two children. Ruth Anne Criswell is his little sister and seven years separate them.

My family includes my Mom, Dad, two sisters and I. Diana Lynn Criswell was born February 3, 1958 in Havre de Grace, Maryland. Deneen Louise Criswell was born October 25, 1964 in Jefferson City, Tennessee. Our initials were all DLC. I was a fairly healthy child other than the croup. The worst episode was when I was about 2 years old. I could not breathe very well, and after being rushed to Dr. Taylor's office where Mrs. Taylor carried me to the shower to sit in the steam for awhile, Dr. Taylor rushed us to the hospital speeding through the toll barrier. Needless to say I survived!

The farm carries so many special memories for me. Nee Nee was a hard worker and quite the cook. She was a very elegant farmer's wife, kept a spotless house, and could prepare a memorable feast. The meal was loaded with multiple dishes of farm fresh food, and family meals were always fun. I was able to enjoy her delicious cooking well into my forties, as my grandmother lived a long life. There was nothing any better than her fried tomatoes and corn fritters for a perfect summer lunch, as I enjoyed many good times with her over the years. My favorite surprise was when there was a rice pudding or maybe a lemon sponge pie in the refrigerator. I have compiled many of her recipes for my use after inheriting her cookbooks, and use them often, but never with that same ability.

Other than the farm, most of my early childhood memories come from Zion, Maryland, where we lived until I was 10 years old. Zion was a close knit little village where we children practically had the run of the town. Only Mr. Allen's yard was off limits! We had a large yard and it was the gathering place for football, softball and general pandemonium. Michael Owens and Steve Foster were often part of the gang of kids that joined us for ball games. Whenever possible, my Dad joined our games. Often a ball would roll into Mr. Allen's yard across the street and go under his hedge. Only the bravest of the moment would dare to crawl under the hedge to retrieve the ball. We had no choice because we didn't have that many balls. We had heard the stories about Mr. Allen not liking children, but I do not recall one encounter.

Our house in Zion had a living room, dining room, kitchen, play room, bathroom and two bedrooms upstairs. Lynn and I shared a bedroom. It had two windows. One was a dormer. We shared a double bed which often caused problems. The bed was pressed under a slanted ceiling and, if we did not settle down after been tucked in bed, Mom or Dad would come in and use the "stick" from the window shade to spank us. They broke many "sticks" too, I might add!

If we were not playing in the big yard with other kids, we were riding our bikes. It was such fun, especially when we played cops and robbers or hide and seek all through the upper side of the village. Crossing the intersection in front of the store was off limits, because there could be a car traveling through. Christy Gambill, my best friend, lived next door. The only problem was that she was not a tomboy like me. So we would make deals. I would suffer through "dolls" for a few hours (or minutes if possible), and she would suffer through football or softball for as long as I could stretch it, or she would send her brothers to play and she stayed home. I do not think I was real nice to Christy many times. She did like to ride bikes and play church. Playing church took place on rainy days in the garage. The stepladder was the organ and an old wooden box was the pulpit. Christy and Lynn took turns playing the organ and piano while I was the preacher. I could preach quite a sermon! In the lower part of the yard we had multiple chestnut trees. Chestnuts were great for eating or throwing, the latter of the two always got us in trouble. We had a hammock tied between two of the trees.

There were several boys in the neighborhood that like to play ball with me. One such fellow was Larry. One evening most other children had gone home, but Larry hung around. Mom and Dad were getting ready for an ice cream social at church with other young adults. Lynn and I were to go to Mom Mom and Pop Pop Clark's for the evening. But I did my best to mess up the evening. Larry and I were playing and I wrapped myself up in the hammock. He began to swing me around like a jump rope. After a few revolutions, I fell out, and as I went to the house crying, he ran home. It was days before we saw Larry again. Mom removed my t-shirt much to my dislike and realized something must be broken. They took me once again to Dr. Taylor's in Rising Sun, Maryland. He was just ready to leave the house himself as we pulled in the driveway. He examined me and said it was a broken collarbone so off to the hospital we headed. Mom and Dad did make it to at least part of the social as I lay on the couch at Mom Mom's house. I remember several days that followed on a bed in the playroom flat on my back. The contraption was quite interesting, and it seemed as if it stayed on forever. But all finally healed and life went back to normal, except the missing Larry who eventually reappeared.

Also, exciting days were happening as Maryland Route 272 was being built from Calvert to North East, Maryland. The bank that was formed during construction provided a great sledding hill either on the snow with a sled or the grass with a piece of cardboard. Watching all the large equipment at work was entertaining.

Down the street from us lived a family that had two girls and we liked to play together sometimes. Their names were Sharon and Charlotte. They had a big brother, Michael, who had little to do with us as we played. Michael did come to my birthday party one year and hung around our yard at times. One summer, we girls had a circus in the Owens' backyard. Each of us had a stunt to perform and we "sold" tickets. No big kids allowed! Another summer the Owens' had a large hornets' nest in a tree in their front yard that hung over the street. A great act of bravery was to ride your bike under that nest and come back again without being stung. I have a few pictures that include Michael during those early years. There are also several pictures of Steve Foster and me as little children. The result of those early friendships definitely stayed woven throughout my life.

When I look back, I guess we were a very typical family of the 50's. Dad worked up the street at the garage for Edgar Thompson. Alfred Owens also worked there. It is strange how life works sometimes as our lives crossed with the Owens' in those early years. Mom stayed at home and took care of us kids, the house, and Dad. We had dinner together every night. Mom was a great cook, too, as she had learned from one of the best. There were certain times that were mealtimes and you had better be there, on time, with hands washed. We ate our vegetables, even the peas, as I covered them with ketchup, said please and thank you, and said our prayers before going to bed. We had a swing set in the backyard and a few trees to climb, along with a little pool for those hot summer days. I can remember getting upset with my friends for getting grass in the pool. For some reason I did not like pieces of grass sticking to me when I was "swimming".

Not to worry, we were not perfect. And for all those imperfections we actually got spankings, sometimes with a stick or belt. And yes, we even heard those dreaded words, "wait until your father gets home." Dad had a way a taking care of things. I have told him there are two things about which I hold a grudge. First, he ran over my hoola hoop with the lawn mower because I left it laying in the yard, and he never replaced it. We were told to always pick up our stuff at the end of the day and put it away. Second, he would not go back for my pinwheel that blew out the car window. He claims he told me not to hold it out so far, because if it went out he would not go back. He was true to his word! Lynn had sense enough to bring her pinwheel back in the car after the warning, but I just had to push the limits.

Mom always made our birthdays special. Even when it was just us, Mom and Dad would sing to us. Dad has never been able to stay on tune, but Mom can and we still enjoy a song over the phone through the years as Dad's off key voice is a treat. I guess that is why I carry on the tradition with favorite meals and a special plate, (the plate is used for a variety of special occasions), and calling anyone in the family on their birthday and singing to them. Mom would prepare us our favorite meal, and we celebrated for the entire day. My favorite meal was usually spaghetti. In our home, Lynn and I knew we were loved. I also realize my parents were very young. My friends through all those growing up years thought my Daddy was quite the handsome guy. People are trained for every other area of life but parenting, but I think my parents were pretty smart. We were surrounded by so much family and a good church, so the wisdom of others was a positive factor.

Life in the small town of Zion, Maryland, was good. We knew everybody and everybody knew us. All it had was one main street, one intersection, the garage, corner store, two churches, and houses of people. Special people stand out. There was Hook and Freda who lived next door. They liked us! There were the Thompson's who owned the garage. We called them "E" and "Yerkie". They were like another set of grandparents to us. They had the coolest house in town. It was quite fancy for our little town with a garage and automatic door opener that housed a fancy car. They had an enclosed porch and the kitchen was unique with a booth area for the kitchen table. Those red padded seats stand out. They had a kitchen clock like a cat, and one day we got one, too. They had ponies, and we got to ride them often. E had a sleigh that he got out in the winter and we rode through the street in snow, and in the summer he had a cart. Christmas mornings for the years while we lived in Zion, they came to our house. E brought his movie camera and set it up as Lynn and I came down the stairs. Christmas morning meant "bright lights" in our eyes. Zion was a great village of people. The Gambills, the Scotts (providing many children to play with), the Dollengers (Earla made Lynn and I a black baby doll that we both still have today), Touchtons (one of them owned the store), Prettymans, the DeMonds, the Fosters, the Thompsons, and, of course, the Owens' would name a few of the Zion families.

I had a pet when we lived in Zion. It was a collie dog whose name was Lady. Lady was a fun and loving dog. I can still remember all that hair! The day we had to give her away before we moved was a day I will not forget. I am jumping ahead, but wanted to tell about our dog. Daddy had borrowed a truck, and we were taking Lady to her new home. Daddy stopped at Campbell's store outside the town of Rising Sun. Lady took advantage of the stop and leapt out of the back of the truck and started running. The last we saw her she was heading for a farm across the road and ran out past the pond. We never found Lady that day. I like to think that someone took her in and cared for her. These events made me sad.

I attended Calvert Elementary School. In my mind, it was quite a large and beautiful brick building. The playground was wonderful and full of trees. School was different in those days. Snow rarely canceled school, and I did not walk to and from school uphill for miles in rain or snow, but the buses did run with chains. The rules were strict, even on the bus, and we obeyed or suffered the consequences. We rode the bus from Zion Garage where Dad worked and I was surrounded by friends, but I hated school. You see, Lynn got to spend her days at home with Mom, hanging around the garage, or being with Yerkie or Nee Nee while I had to go to school. My early school days were not pleasant as I clearly did not want to be there. For reasons not known, I was extremely insecure! In those days there was no kindergarten, so I went directly to first grade and I think I missed the fun part of starting school. Mrs. Reynolds was my teacher, and she was a nice lady, but I was very unhappy. I sure gave Mom plenty of trouble about going to school for the first few weeks, and then I settled in. Second grade was better in my memory. Mrs. Gifford was my teacher, and she and I got along quite well. Third grade was Mrs. Mason, and she was also a very loving teacher. If I had a rough start that year, I don't remember. But fourth grade was a different story. Enter into my life, Mrs. Kelly. Now you need to know that she loved my Dad when he was in school. He was her pet. But she did not really like girls, especially problem girls, and I am sure my reputation followed me. She had a hard-nosed way of running the classroom. You were seated according to your grades and attendance. Now I was not a bad student, but there were others much smarter. Christy Gambill, my best friend, was one of them, along with Robbie England, Art Newman and Gary Mink. They were always seated first. The order changed, but it was always them. The poor guys in the back of the room I felt sorry for, but worried more about me, usually seated in the middle. Every time grades came out, I hoped my position would improve. Then if you got sick, you returned to find yourself in the rear of the classroom. There was the day we saw a barn fire in Rising Sun, Maryland, on the way home from church. I went in the next day to tell Mrs. Kelly, she yelled at me for being out so late at night, and did not want to hear my story. There is one good memory from her class...eating tapioca pudding. She would have us try new things, and this one I liked. One day I finally cracked. I refused to go to school. What a mess Mom had on her hands. The majority of my lifetime spankings came during the beginning of fourth grade. They spent time with the principal and tried to work it out. Even the principal thought I was just a spoiled brat. I was finally put into another class. They had a second class that was fourth and fifth combined. Maybe God was getting me ready for teaching in a small school even then. What a disaster for a teacher. This teacher would fall asleep on a regular basis. I am not sure what I learned that year, but Mrs. Kelly was out of my life. I wrapped up that time period rather easily here on paper, but for my parents it must have been a long difficult year. Any problems I have today, I blame on those early school years. This did not end my school problems. There will be more about school later in the story.

Family was important to us. We spent much time with grandparents and extended family, and from them I leaned many things. Nee Nee's family, Uncle Arthur and Aunt Helen (her sister)that allowed us to spend time in the Newark area playing with cousins. Add to them our time with Ruth, my grandmothers' sister, Cliff, Lanny and Joy over the years. Those days on the farm bring smiles today. I was young enough to enjoy all the fun stuff of farming without the hard work. Playing in the hayloft was probably my favorite. Our city cousins (whose mom, Aunt Margaret, Pop Pop's sister-in-law, would make them wear their suits on Sunday and not get dirty) would come for long visits in the summer and we had a great time together. There was Uncle Joe (the doctor) and Aunt Mary, Uncle Walter, who spent much time with me playing store and Aunty Beck, who was well endowed, and Bill Criswell, whom I affectionately called Bully. Bully and I spent lots of time together when they would visit the farm. We would go for long walks and I always knew the way home. These cousins were actually Dad and Ruthie's first cousins. The most fun were Janice and Dave. They were full of energy and made me happy. Nee Nee loved to cook for all the family. I know I already told you how good a cook she was, but some things are worth mentioning again. Those pies, cookies, and cakes were delicious and she was always cooking something. Almost until the day she went to heaven, she cooked as if cooking for farm hands. Gathering eggs with Nee Nee was my least favorite job. Those chicken lice just waited for me and jumped on every time. Pop Pop taught me many things besides the feel of an electric fence, though quite memorable! I also can still feel his hand squeezing my leg, especially when we were sitting at the table for meals even after I was grown. He taught me to drive the tractor and attempted to teach me to back up a wagon. He was such a hard worker and milked all those cows daily with very few breaks. He taught me about milking, and if I opened my mouth wide he could hit it with some fresh warm milk straight from the cow. He could do that with the barn cats, too. The best watermelon you ever ate was on the farm, good and cold straight out of the milk cooler. The best corn was fresh corn on canning day when the kitchen was piled high with corn on the cob, and I got to suck the cobs after the corn was cut off by many helping hands. We then carried the cobs to those waiting chickens.

Ruthie is such a part of the farm memories. She is eleven years older than I am and has always been a part of my life. I still have a little baby doll that I named "Wake Up Little Susie" because she taught me to sing that song from the Everly Brothers. She was a great example of how to be a tomboy. She later married Donald Thomas and I have three cousins, Dale, Craig and Kerry. We shared many times together with Nee Nee, Pop Pop, and the family. Ruthie is such a big part of my life to this day. Her energy is contagious and I can only hope to grow older as gracefully. I always enjoy the time I spend with her. She can cook like her mother! Ruthie is known for her ability to ask questions. She will find out what she wants to know! We all laugh when Ruthie ask you a question about the person seated beside her instead of directly asking that person. She had learned that from her mother. When our sons, Darrell and Jared, entered the picture, (which made Ruthie very happy) they affectionately called her "Roo Roo". She always waved goodbye with two hands. We still call her "Roo" and she usually remembers to wave with two hands.

The layout and furnishings of the farmhouse and barn are still in my memory. How I wish that when the farm was sold, I would have been old enough to have had some of those furnishings. The giant kitchen and large table, the dining room with the wall cupboards, and table and chairs and old desk are still vivid. The phone in the corner was another memory. In those days we had the old party lines. Several people were on one line. You heard every ring, but knew if it was your ring by the sound. For example, your ring may be one long and two shorts. I guess it made for some interesting times as others could listen in on your conversations. The wraparound porch with the outside basin also stands out and Nee Nee sure kept it clean. Scrubbing the porch was a regular duty. Good memories come from the farm.

Traveling to Conowingo, Maryland, actually Rowlandsville, along Basin Run Creek with the Octoraro Creek down at the bottom of the hill, we would visit Mom Mom and Pop Pop Clark. To give you a perspective on the map, the Octoraro Creek spills into the Susquehanna River just south of the Conowingo Dam, which dumps into the Chesapeake Bay and flows on to the Atlantic Ocean. The sound of the creek always made for great sleeping. Mom Mom, also, was a great cook. Her fried chicken and mashed potatoes were the best. She made great iced tea, but it always had "dirt" in the bottom of the pitcher and glass because she made her tea from loose tea leaves. If you drank it slowly, you could make the leaves stay on the last half inch of the tea. Mom Mom had a green thumb and a love for flowers. She taught me to love them also. I spent many hours with her in the flower and vegetable gardens learning the names of plants, pulling weeds and reaping the harvest. Today my flower garden still produces Irises and Bachelor Buttons transplanted from her garden. I also enjoy growing a few vegetables such as tomatoes, cucumbers, green beans and hot peppers as a result of my grandmothers' influences. Mom Mom loved house plants, too. In the winter, one of the bedrooms upstairs was filled with potted plants. We always said we were sleeping in a funeral home if we spent the night. A full moon on a winter's night could make strange shadows in the room. My eyes would watch them until they could stay open no longer. We also had many snake stories from her house. I think it was snake haven. If it was baseball season, Pop Pop could be found listening to an Orioles ballgame on the radio in the kitchen or watching the game, if it was televised. He introduced me (only visually) to soft shelled crabs. I have vivid memories of him eating them between two slices of bread with legs hanging out and eyes looking at you. I have never gotten the nerve to try them. Mealtimes at their house were very interesting. Pop Pop did not believe you should talk at the table. Mealtime was eating time and nothing else. He did loosen up as we grew and allowed us to talk but he always ate quietly at the table. I loved my grandparents, even if I was a little afraid of Pop Pop Clark.

Aunt Kay and Uncle Clarence were such a big part of our lives. We spent so much time with them and my three guy cousins, Dennis, Kenny and Ronnie, during all my growing up years. They had a cabin at Broad Creek north of the Conowingo Dam on the Susquehanna River. We spent many a summer day there boating, skiing, swimming (dropping into the creek from the rope swing) and spending time together. Meals together were special times and we always enjoyed Aunt Kay's potato salad along with many games we played as families. Family reunions with Mom Mom and clan were quite memorable. I especially enjoyed the day of playing softball and Mom Mom pulled Aunt Kay's shorts down as she was running bases. There is more than one way to win a ballgame! Many good family memories were made with the Clark family.

Uncle Ben was a part of my life at my grandparents' house, and our house in Zion and later in Tennessee, as he would come and spend time with us. Ben was also instrumental later in my life through a job offer. The list of Mom's brothers and sisters in order is Freddie who married Ruth and had two sons, Michael and Mark, Mom, Kay who married Uncle Clarence with three sons, Dennis, Kenny and Ronnie, Mary Ellen who married Bob with two children, Melanie and Kevin, and Ben who married Jan with two children, Jonathan and Lindsay. Ben is four years older than I am, so he did let me hang out with him sometimes. I think only because I was cheap entertainment. The list of things he has done to me is quite long, but I must tell a few. He shot me with a BB gun in my backside. On purpose, too, I might add. He would take me for long walks and check to see if I was paying attention and make me lead us home. I did get better at that little game. One day on our walk, we went across the railroad bridge. In the middle of the bridge he got down to listen and said a train was coming and we needed to hang over the side as there was not enough time to reach the other end. As I began to climb over the railing, he changed his mind. I guess he cared a little. One other time when we were playing in Basin Run up near the waterfall, I stepped on a can lid and cut open my toe. That day he carried me all the way home. Maybe they all balance out!

As I mentioned, I was a tomboy and really enjoyed the outdoors the most. Bath time proved that as Mom would scrub my legs very hard to get them clean only to realize she was trying to scrub off the bruises. We did have a TV with rabbit ears for increased reception, and I enjoyed Captain Kangaroo, Sally Star, and Romper Room. As I got older, shows like Sky King, I Love Lucy, and Wyatt Earp were among my favorites. If it was possible, my day was spent outdoors playing with my Zion friends. Daddy liked to play ball with us, too. He could throw a ball the hardest and kick a football the highest of anyone in the world.

We attended and were very active in the church at Conowingo. It was quite a long drive, I thought, and Lynn and I spent the time either singing or fighting. I think Mom and Dad preferred the singing. There were many influences there in my life, the greatest being our pastor, Walter Burcham. We spent time at the Burcham's house, too. I can still hear his voice as he preached. I did listen. The music also stands out in my mind. Mom sang in a sextet along with two of her sisters and three others. The choir was excellent. Mom would bring raisins to church for my snack and if I was tired, I could lay my head against her and she would tickle my arm. I still like to have my arm tickled. Those ceilings seemed so high and those marble looking lights seemed quite large. I have such good memories of Sunday School at Conowingo. Mrs. Funk was my beginner teacher and her love for us was apparent in all she did. Mom and Dad were growing rapidly under Pastor Burcham and if the doors were open we were there. I learned much about Jesus during that time in my life and as a little girl I talked to Mom about Jesus. We sat on the front porch swing and I asked Jesus to come into my heart and be a part of my life. Not exactly sure what that meant to me that day, although I did believe that God sent his Son, Jesus, to die for my sins and I knew what sin was by that time in my life. I believe God heard the prayer of that little five year old girl and is keeping His Word to complete the work He began that day. Later, during my teaching years, a special student brought a gift of a miniature porch swing after I had told my swing story to my students. Those early teachings and understandings were important to my spiritual growth. Because of what God was doing in Mom and Dad's lives, our entire family life was about the change. Looking back, I would not trade the next chapter of my life for anything, even though at the time, it was the hardest thing in the world for our family to do.

So many early childhood memories surrounded the times with my grandparents. I remember the feeling of being loved, cuddled, and even spoiled by my grandmothers. The family times were the best... like sitting under a large tree enjoying the shade and a glass of milk, Kool-Aid, or iced tea, a cookie, and feeling very secure. Likewise, today, I want my grandchildren to know of my unconditional love for each of them and remember the best times did not come from things, but are products of the time I can give them along their journey. I love my family. No strings attached. Childhood circles often go unnoticed when you are a kid, but looking back I am grateful for them all.

Zephaniah 3:17 NKJV
"The Lord your God in your midst, The Mighty One, will save; He will rejoice over you with gladness, He will quiet you with His love, He will rejoice over you with singing."

No matter where life may take you, there is something to be learned and some treasure from the experiences to carry through your life. The hardest of times will teach you the most lasting lessons, and hard times are certain to come. As I watch my family grow, my mom side wants to protect them from all the bumps, bruises and bangs of life, but experience shows these are our growing points. The previous verse reminds me of where God is at all times in our lives. He is in the middle of my circles.

Chapter 2

Journey to Tennessee

The first memory I have of big changes about to occur in our family is seeing Mom and Dad seated cross-legged on their bedroom floor facing each other. They had called Lynn and me into the room, and by their body language something big was in the wind. Slowly, they began to talk to us and Dad told us that "God had called him to preach". Now I am not exactly sure what that meant to a ten year old, and I am not certain I remember. But the ramifications of that discussion began to sink in over the next few weeks as we prepared to move to Jefferson City, Tennessee, for Dad to attend college. Now I think I have just painted a picture of the "perfect" childhood in Zion. I have certainly shown you how much I loved my grandparents, and now my little mind is whirling trying to comprehend leaving it all. All the details that come with being an adult were the least of my worries. I do not remember selling the house, but I do remember loading the truck. I really do not remember saying goodbye to everyone, but I do remember the feeling of being so homesick for my family in Maryland. There was no going back for any of us. Lynn and I were in this together, but until now we had never done anything well when we were in it together!

I do remember arriving in Jefferson City. Obviously Dad had prepared for us to arrive, and our new house was ready for us to move into immediately. It was on a side street near Carson Newman College. It was more like a half house or an apartment, and there were many other half houses surrounding us filled with other college students and their families. I remember what seemed to me as a very large basically white rock protruding from the front yard. This is also the land of cockroaches. I learned about those ugly things, and when Mom would bring home groceries, Lynn and I would empty the bags on the porch as to not bring any roaches into the house. The bathroom wall had a hole so large that, from the bathtub, you could see the railroad tracks out back, and Daddy had to repair that one. There was no more giant backyard to play in, or any friends running to greet me on that day. Lynn and I could only stand to be together for so long and finally I went looking for another playmate. Carrying one item I was comfortable with, my football, I stood in the backyard leaning against the clothesline pole when a boy walked up. Johnny asked if I knew how to throw that thing, and I quickly demonstrated my ability. We became friends that day, and so began my new life. I recall the homesickness we all felt for many weeks as we adjusted. People from Maryland would send us letters and that was exciting, but when someone was coming to visit, now that was the best news ever.

I know Daddy struggled with some of his classes as he had not been in school for some time now, and he would get into big theological discussions with some of the professors. Often on Sunday we would have roasted professor for dinner. But Daddy never quit. He worked hard and somehow there was always enough. I am still not sure how that happened sometimes, but God always supplied. So much about the day-to-day functions of our house was way over my head, but looking back I know it could not have been easy. There is something lasting to be learned by not being handed it all as a child, but I had no idea we had so little.

And oh the homesickness, oh yes, I did mention that, didn't I? But it stands out. I remember that first Christmas we could not afford to go to Maryland so Mom and Dad did their best to make it a good one. Now Christmas was always a special time for me and most of my memories were not about the gifts, but family. Gifts had always been held to a minimum with us usually receiving one big gift. The gifts didn't change that year, but the family was sure missing. So this year, Mom decorated that tree in her traditional blue lights with blue and silver balls, fixed a great meal, and we tried, but I know everyone was so glad when that day was over. Mom and Dad made friends quickly and we would spend time with other people often who were in the same situation and far from home. I am sure glad I grew up in a family that loves people.

I started school at Jefferson City Elementary School. Now remember, school is not my favorite thing. I do not remember any great trauma in fifth and sixth grade, but I do remember worrying that Daddy would forget to pick us up sometimes, not like he had ever forgotten before. If he was late, I would panic. Lynn always remained calm. I knew he was a busy man. I must have been a pain of a child worrying about so many things that were the adult worries not mine. I must have done most of my worrying as a child because as an adult I really do not worry about things excessively, although my insecurities still lingered into adulthood.

The biggest memory is sixth grade. It was November 22, 1963. My class was on the playground and Mrs. Dryer called to us from the classroom window. She told us we needed to come inside because she had something to tell us, and we could all tell she was very sad. Of course, that day we heard the news that President Kennedy had been shot. Everyone was so sad for a long time. I will always remember that day at the window.

Another life changing event happened in Jefferson City, Tennessee. One day Mom and Dad told Lynn and I we were about to have a new little baby born into the family. That was exciting news! Oh how I wanted a brother named David. But…Deneen arrived instead. Now I would not trade her for anything and I am certainly thankful for all the nieces and nephews she has given me, but she was kind of spoiled! Supposedly Lynn and I were responsible for that. After all, I was 12 years older than she was and she became more fun when she could finally do something, but until then we carried her way too much. The day she was born we could not go into the hospital. Daddy took Lynn and me for a visit and lifted us up to the window to wave to Mom. Getting a new little sister was the best thing that happened in Tennessee! She sure brightened up our lives. Another good thing happened when she was born. Nee Nee arrived by train to Jefferson City to help out around the house, so we were able to spend time with our Grandmother!

By now I was getting very comfortable with the neighborhood and enjoying my friends. One of our favorite pastimes was hanging out in the tall grass beside the road with an old purse tied with a string. We would place the purse in the street, and people would stop and back up as we reeled in the purse. It went well for awhile until we were caught and reported to our parents. Grownups always spoil fun!

Now again life as I knew it was about to change. A little church out in the sticks asked Daddy to come and be their Pastor. I remember that drive to visit. As we drove down the winding dirt road, the sights are forever etched in my brain. Some very poor people with very few nice things lived along this road. The church at New Blackwell, Rutledge, Tennessee, was a picturesque white church building on a hillside, steeple reaching toward the sky, with a fenced cemetery next door, and surrounded by tobacco fields. Long story short, Daddy said yes, and for a while we commuted from Jefferson City. We eventually moved into the parsonage they built just for us and were the only ones around with indoor plumbing. The Satterfields lived in a shack not far from us and their little girl came one day and actually took a bath at our house. It was her first bath in an indoor tub. The house we lived in was a mansion compared to any around us. The Croxdales lived next door and became good friends. They owned a horse, a Tennessee Walker, and we got to ride him sometimes. I even learned to top tobacco in their field, as tobacco was one of their top money making crops. It is hard work!

Many special people came into our lives at New Blackwell. Mrs. Moore was the first one. Her husband was Daddy's first funeral, and she became another grandmother to us. She lived just over on the ridge from our house, she made us clothes, and we visited her often. Another special family was the Kidwells. They owned a farm about two ridges over and we spent many days at their place. Farm life was familiar to me and being there was comfortable. Like my farming grandmother back home, Aileen Kidwell could cook. She made the best homemade biscuits. Sometimes it felt like being back at Nee Nee's or Mom Mom's house again.

Now as the parsonage took a little while to finish, we stayed in Jefferson City for the rest of sixth grade and then moved to the country before seventh grade. God and Dad had a way of always moving us during the summer so changing schools was not so dramatic. But nothing could prepare me for this change. During the summer we helped around the parsonage, and I tended to explore a little too much. One day I stepped on a nail and had to be taken to the nearest doctor for a tetanus shot. That doctor was in Rutledge and let it suffice to say it is a miracle I did not die of some dread disease picked up in that dirty place. We moved into our new house with great excitement. These country folks were different from people I knew back home. The men sat on one side of the church and the women on the other side. Then there was a very large lady who needed to sit over a brace on the pew to keep from breaking it. There were the sweet Greenlees who would do anything for us. Sorry we never got to know the Hatfield's or McCoy's.

We did have many visitors from Maryland during our years in Tennessee. Dad was ordained as a minister at New Blackwell, and that brought many people from home. Being raised in a home that loved people, guests were not unusual. Also, we lived close to Gatlinburg and the Great Smoky Mountains, and with the exception of the Gambills because the brakes went out in our car in Pigeon Forge, we took them all to the mountains for a day. People like Peggy and Earl and the girls, Aunt Kay, Uncle Clarence and the boys, Uncle Ben, and so many other family and friends enjoyed the beauty of the mountains while visiting us. I always enjoyed stopping at "Hillbilly Village" for the cherry cider. When Ruthie and Donald came to visit, Ruthie walked up Clingman's Dome in the mountains while quite pregnant. We would see many bear, sometimes with their cubs, and usually spent time in the cold creek that winded through the mountains.

Each fall, while we resided in East Tennessee, our family would go to Gatlinburg to spend a couple of nights. We always stayed in a motel with a heated pool. I have such good memories of playing together on those vacations. The cost, we later learned, was $12.00 per night, and we finally understood how hard it was as Dad saved a few dollars during those years for us to have this vacation.

Money was an issue, even though I really had no idea we were poor. Daddy made $30.00 per week pastoring the church while attending college and paying household expenses. Mom was a wise spender, and I never realized we wore handmade clothing because of cost. I thought we were just stylish! I do remember cupboards being rather empty, but did not know it should be otherwise. I do not remember going hungry. Mom always had meals on the table at mealtime. So often we would go to the mailbox and find a letter from someone back home with money inside. I saw firsthand how God would supply when we had a need. Mom told me of one day when a letter contained a ten dollar bill. She was so excited, because it bought me a new pair of sneakers as mine were full of holes, a gallon of milk and a ham bone to add to the beans she already had for soup. Maybe Lynn even got something, and Mom could save a couple of dollars for another day. I loved Mom's bean soup. I thought that was why we ate it so often. Our cupboards were never full. When I look at our pantry today it is hard to imagine opening that door only to see some crackers, maybe peanut butter and a few canned goods. Again some good lessons and cause to realize how much I take for granted today. Remember to keep a grateful heart for the little things.

Now you have already figured out that school is an issue with me. It only gets worse for the next two years. I entered seventh grade and Lynn entered third grade in a two room schoolhouse complete with outhouses and a coal stove for heating. In the next two years, the only education I got at school was functioning in a classroom with fifth through eighth graders in one room. Actually, I taught most of the class how to tell time and helped them memorize the multiplication tables. The only part I enjoyed was playing ball at recess or going to the woods to collect kindling for the fire. The schoolhouse was down the hill from the church and we walked the short distance to and from school. If the circumstances got out of hand, running home was always an option. I did do that on two occasions. One occasion was merited and the other was not. Just being sick of school was not a reason to run away from school in Dad's eyes. The bus driver and our teacher in a fist fight out front of the school was a good reason. Our parents tried to move us to a different school, but the county said no. They were not positive years at school, and did not help me to like school any better, but made for some good stories. Later when I would tell my students about my two room schoolhouse experiences, they all thought I was a well-preserved 90 year old!

Home was where I wanted to be most of the time or at the neighbors helping with farm chores, picking persimmons in season, and riding their horse. Dad hung a tire in the tree in our front yard and taking my lessons from Johnny Unitas, I practiced until I could thread that tire with my football while it was swinging. I had just gotten a new football for my birthday which I happened to find a few days early hidden in the chest freezer in the basement. Now exactly how a thirteen year old girl was to use this skill was yet to be seen. Perhaps it was so I could "wow" my fifth and sixth grade boys later as the teacher who could actually play all time quarterback at recess!

We did make several trips back and forth to Maryland watching Interstate 81 being built. Dad would get excited every time a new piece was finished. I think they completed that road the year we moved back to Maryland. One Christmas, we did not travel home and the temperature reached 70 degrees and no one felt like it was Christmas. We decided just to pretend it wasn't, as if that would help. One trip home we surprised everyone by showing up. I remember arriving at the farm in the middle of the night, and Dad held me up so I could knock on Pop and Nee Nee's bedroom window to wake them. I am glad they had a bedroom on the first floor of the farmhouse by then. Pop Pop got so excited and yelled, "Mildred, its Donnie!"

Many good family times and good people are a result of our years at New Blackwell. I learned to drive our VW Beetle around the church during those years. I fell in love with Krispy Crème Donuts, especially when the "HOT" sign was on, while living in Tennessee. As I said earlier, I would not trade those years if I could. Watching my Dad graduate was a great example of how God provides for us, and how hard work paid off. God had taken care of us through some hard years and formed another circle that would not be forgotten. Again, I am grateful for the people on my journey.

Now another part of the journey was about to begin. We were moving! Perhaps I block out goodbyes, but once again I do not remember leaving Tennessee, but I was ready to be back in good ole Maryland. Change is not my favorite thing, but I was ready or so I thought for this one.

A note to my sons and families…Always take time for your family. Now I am not talking about your parents (even though I know you will always take time for us), but I am referring to your own families. Be careful not to spend every chance to get away visiting extended family. Build those bonds strong with your children by spending vacation time with your spouse and children. Explore new places. Day trips will teach you local history and you never know what you may find in some corner of your world. You will create memories that children will always remember. Memories come in unexpected ways. The little things are so important. Time is the essential ingredient and time does not stand still.

Chapter 3

Journey Back to Maryland

Just as a reminder, it is 1966. I am thirteen years old and will be fourteen in December. I am about to enter the ninth grade...high school. I was scared to death. We just left the sticks and were coming to the big town of North East, Maryland. I had five fellow students in my eighth grade class and now there is one hundred. Most people would still laugh at this amount, but I was overwhelmed. Quite an increase!

We had been gone from Maryland for four years, and there were many changes. The biggest change was Nee Nee and Pop Pop Criswell had sold the farm and built a house on the corner of the property. Pop Pop missed the farm until the day he died. Mom Mom and Pop Pop Clark still lived in Rowlandsville for now. We were moving into another house and remember I just wasn't crazy about change. Perhaps by now, I was beginning to understand the circles of friends that were accumulating in my life.

We moved into a farmhouse on Warburton Road that would be my home for the next almost four years. Dad was now the Pastor of a church in North East, Maryland. It was time to make more new friends at home, church and school. I was not thrilled at the prospect and became even more bashful for a period of time as my insecurities flourished. The good part about it all is that we were back in Maryland surrounded by extended family. Back to the dinners at Nee Nee's with Ruthie and gang, back to Mom Mom's, Aunt Kay's and the adventures at their houses, enjoying time with cousins again.

During these years, we went on a couple of great vacations. Somehow, I never saw us as campers, but we did a couple of camping trips on our own and with Aunt Kay, Uncle Clarence and boys. I sure remember the Canada trip when I woke up with a very swollen face from mosquitoes. I also remember the time we used our friends, the Hudlers, truck camper and Dad ended up on Madison Avenue in New York City driving a camper! Lynn and I were glad we were in the back and not anywhere near Dad as he maneuvered out of that situation. Mom and Deneen were sitting in the cab and I imagine things were slightly tense. Loud burst of temper runs in the family. Beach time with Aunt Kay and the cousins was important during these years, too, as we spent many days in the sun and surf. Best of all, Christmases would be spent with all the family once again. Going from one house to another on Christmas Day, playing games with cousins and eating way too much food was all treasured. We were home!

Let us look at our "new" house. Now it was a working farm we lived on and the house was quite large according to my standards. It did not have that many rooms, but each room was big. Downstairs we had a family room, hallway with stairway and backdoor, kitchen, and living room. Upstairs we had a large end bedroom that would hold twin beds and toys for Lynn and Deneen. For several months that large bedroom also held two other children. Billy and Cathy were two little children that came to live with us and stole our hearts. Their parents were in prison, and for a little while, they became a part of our family.

Giving to others is a characteristic our parents taught us by example. I cannot talk about our home without talking about the people who shared it with us. They were what made it special. So many visitors over the years came to our house. Open your home to others. Do not give only to those who will give back. Find the lonely, the unloved or the ones down because of circumstances and give! My parents taught me to help others when possible and Michael and I do this whenever an opportunity arises. You will also benefit from giving to others.

Now back to the house. Next to that bedroom was the bathroom and then crossing over the stairway landing was my bedroom and down the hall was Mom and Dad's bedroom. The yard was large and there was much to explore. We could even have a dog. Someone gave us Ralph, a puppy of mixed breeds, who ended up having puppies (oops) and we changed her name to Ralphetta.

The best part about the farm was the family from whom we rented the house. Mr. and Mrs. Moore had several children, but the youngest of them were Helen and Eleanor (another friendship that has lasted over the years). Helen was a little older than I and Eleanor a little younger. We spent hours with them. Helen is in heaven now, but our friendship with Eleanor endures time. We practically lived outside, weather permitting, and inside on bad days we played many a card game. Miles Bournes was our favorite card game, but we also enjoyed Pit and Twister. The Moore's had a pony and pony cart that we learned to operate. That pony brought us much joy and disgust depending on his mood. We also rode horses and helped with some farm chores. They had peacocks and we would sell feathers by the side of the road. That business was not real successful, but I did master the peacock call. In the backyard was an old chicken house that we renovated for a cabin and quite the cabin it was. It slept 5-6 people and we carried more food to that place than 20 people could eat. If only we all kept our rooms as neatly as we kept that cabin. The property also had a large pond with an island. Mr. Moore even brought in a load of sand to make a beach for us. Summer days always included a swim, and sometimes the St. Bernard, Chris, would join us. He would put his paws on your shoulders and push you under the water. We had a row boat, and one day I as was helping Helen haul the mower out to mow the island; we flipped the mower out of the boat. I do not think that mower ever dried out enough to be used again.

Winter would bring the snow and sledding on the big front hill. We had a toboggan and sleds, but the best was the year we had a car hood. We could pile many people on that hood and fly down the hill sometimes going under the barbed wire fence to the creek. In one sledding accident, I did break my nose and that was not the last time it was broken. We also sledded on the road when the snows were deep. One day we begged the snowplow driver not to plow the hill. I even lay down in the road to stop him. After insisting that I move, he plowed anyway, so we went back to the field to sled. My favorite thing in the winter snows was riding with Dad in the old Desoto. We called it the Buffalo and we could push snow over the hood and still keep moving. Winter also meant some snow days with no school. In those days they put chains on the buses and school went on unless it was really deep. Mom would make homemade donuts on a snow day! If my parents could have confined me to that farm for the next four years, life would have been easier for us all. There are so many good family memories in that farmhouse.

Somehow when you are a kid you think time will stand still, but we all must grow up sometime. One hard memory while living there was the death in a car accident of Frank Graybeal, one of Dad's best friends and the owner of Calvert Manor Nursing Home. We all learn that death is a part of life. Home was the haven in which I could hide from the world. But North East High School was about to enter my life.

Oh, how I hate new schools, new friends, new surroundings and most of all, new teachers. Teachers and I do not have a happy history. So here we go again, but this time to high school. Ninth grade meant each class in a different room and a different teacher. Not only was changing classes difficult, but so was finding my way around the high school, remembering where my locker was, plus the combination, and trying to remember names. Now some names make an impression, and Emily Baker Cameron Morris was one of those. She was my ninth grade Algebra teacher and so often her initials were on the board under math problems and these words, "Do Not Erase, EBCM". Memory is a strange ability. That first year at NEHS I remained very shy and it took a while to make friends.

I was at a new high school as well as a new church, with many opportunities to make friends which I eventually did. Ginny Buchanan became my best friend at school and soon Cindy (Lee) Foster would enter my life through church and become my best friend for life. Ginny was living in Florida, and we reconnected in recent years, but she suddenly became ill with pancreatic cancer and passed away the summer of 2011. Cindy remains my dear forever friend and I cannot imagine life without her. There are a few others I have connected with again. High school friends generally go in different directions, even though we all thought it would be different with us. Most I do not even know where they are today, but we were friends through it all in high school. The 60's happened around us and not to us. We were affected by the styles and the music, but basically protected from the drug culture of the day. I still have my heavily patched bell bottoms and fringed jacket in the attic.

Spending time with my family doing the little things was always fun. Sometimes after church we would go to the Bar H in North East and get milkshakes and footlong hotdogs. Now Dad would never allow us to eat in the car, as he was rather fanatical about his clean cars. Anyway, I was so shy that I would not order at the window. Even at McDonalds, I would not order food. That shyness was about to change. I think a lot of it is because of where we were until 9th grade. Until North East, my life was basically with my family. Now things were changing. I learned to compensate for my insecurities by becoming a people pleaser. Always trying to please others is not a good choice. Slowly, I was becoming a follower instead of a leader.

Soon, driving became a part of my life so, therefore, did cars! I loved cars… cleaning and driving them and often too fast. A bad habit had emerged, and when our sons were teenagers and we were running late, they always told Dad to let Mom drive. I am also a fanatic about keeping a car clean. I learned that one very well from my Dad. From the engine to the interior down to the wheels and tires, I always want my cars to shine. My favorite color vehicle has been red, from our red Charger to the red Dart and two red Jeeps.

Now, do not think I was the perfect daughter or student once I reached high school. As I expanded my friendships and began to find my way socially at school, I found myself wanting to be with friends more and more. I became bolder and the shy little girl disappeared. I will begin with school. My grades took a hit as I became the social butterfly around school. Suddenly I found myself with many friends and found it too important to please them. We often pushed the limits of especially our vice principal that actually liked us, but found he needed to discipline us at times.

Some events in high school that stand out include the day we staged a riot (remember this is the 60's) between the blacks and the whites. The blacks stood at the bottom of the stairs near the front doors and the whites stood at the top of the stairs near the main office. As we began to yell, I thought the Principal would have a heart attack as he came out of the office. We tried to keep going, but everyone just began to laugh. Our Principal did not think it was too funny, but we all got off easy. Actually, the races got along quite well during those years at NEHS. How thankful I am for this small town high school. We had many advantages being a small, country high school. Another day I was called to the office from class only to find the office staff looking out the front windows laughing. They were enjoying the fact that I was receiving a parking ticket for parking too close to the fire hydrant, when I thought I had squeezed in the open area. Several times, I must admit I would skip class. I had learned my way around the school very well. Also, we knew the back stairs that led to the roof of the school. That was a fun place to go on a beautiful spring day. We would also sneak off school property, through the alley past the water tower (where all the good fights were held), and go to the laundry mat. Now that probably does not sound real exciting, but the laundry mat had vending machines! We would pool our change and carry sodas and candy back into school. Skipping school did get me into trouble many times. One day, of all days, after a friend and I left school to go up the street to her house, a big event took place at school. Someone had called in a bomb scare. My dear Dad, after hearing of the scare, came to school to pick me up and learned I was not there. The report that my Dad had been at school reached me, and I knew grounding was coming. When I did arrive home that day, Mom simply held out her hand in which I placed the car keys. I knew the drill. No car for a month and back to riding the bus.

One other time that I will confess, was when a group of us went to the YMCA to play some volleyball. They had an outdoor court in front of the building along Rt. 40. The problem-it was a school day and Mom happened to drive by and see us all. Mom actually blew the horn, waved, and ruined the rest of my day. When I got home we went through the drill again. I must say, my car got some long periods of rest.

Any more confessions about my high school years and the various activities must be coerced by some type of torture. Some stories about growing up are best to keep only on a need to know basis. Stay away from those old friends, as I am certain their memories have faded over time. Cindy Foster and I have an agreement...so do not bother to question her. I will take some stories to my grave. I am thankful for a God who forgives sin when we ask... past, present and future. His grace, love and mercy are incredible. Scripture teaches us that God casts our sins as far away as the east is from the west.

Speaking again of my car, I did have a few over the years. One was a white Chevy II four door. The only problem, it had a hole in the back floor. My friends learned to be very careful when entering the backseat as to not find your foot on the road! I even had a convertible for a short time, and was known to drive it with the top down and heat blaring in the middle of winter. I loved cars and guys with cool cars were attractive. This was a very shallow reason to find a guy attractive, but the truth. The other car that stands out was my Barracuda. It was baby blue in color with a push button transmission on the dash. It was a 1964 with the long hatch, and I loved that car. When Michael and I started to date, he was driving a 1965 silver, with black stripe, Barracuda, and I always said our cars fell in love first! One time, after I rolled through a stop sign on Wheatly Road, I turned quickly into Zion, went to the garage and switched cars with Michael and pulled back out on the highway as a trooper drove by carefully checking me out. I must admit I drove much too fast and crazy, and only by the grace of God do any of us survive the teenage years. I hope you notice how I turned the fast driving from a story about me to all of you, my readers. Now I am getting ahead of myself. I will back up and get out of high school first.

I have always loved sports as you can already tell, and really enjoy football. My favorite team was the Baltimore Colts, as I already mentioned Johnny U; but I also liked the Green Bay Packers, because playing football in the snow is my idea of the real deal. Oh, yes and I was angry when the Colts were taken in the night from Baltimore, but today I am a Ravens fan. Actually when you think about it, the Ravens name fits Baltimore better than Colts anyway. So get over it people!

Since playing football on a team was out of the question, my next love was basketball. My basketball hero was Pete Maravich. "Pistol Pete" brought new life to a great game. He broke college scoring records at Louisiana State University and played the game with an unbeatable style. Because of Pistol Pete, Converse high tops were a must on the basketball court in the 60's for me and others. Many hours were spent playing basketball at my cousin's house, the Abrams, in Bayview. They lived and breathed basketball. In high school I did not enjoy basketball, because girls still played the old way. There were six players on a team, three played defense, and three played offense. It was slow and boring. By the time I was a junior in high school; the rules for girls changed and were more equal to the boys. During my senior year, I thoroughly enjoyed playing on the team and, also, played field hockey and volleyball and would later play softball on our church team for many years. I am also a baseball fan, enjoying the Baltimore Orioles and the Aberdeen Ironbirds. Sports are a part of me...football, basketball (especially March Madness), and baseball are my three seasons!

By my senior year, I had made my way into the hearts of many of the teachers. Despite my escapades, they liked me. Many of my teachers were fresh out of college, in their first year of teaching, making us close in age. Mr. Wolfe, the biology teacher, who was much older, was probably the toughest teacher I had, but I learned more in his class than any other because he demanded so much more. The teacher who had the greatest impact on my life at school was Mary Etta Reedy. She was my coach for field hockey, basketball and volleyball and became a friend. We spent much time together playing sports, before, during, and after school. If you

wanted to find me before, after or between classes at school, just check the gym. Playing all of those sports helped with my school grades, too. I had to work hard to stay on the teams and Reedy worked us hard to become winners. Mary Etta always called me a "scrappy" player. Sports helped my confidence levels to improve. I really think I was a late bloomer and another year in high school would have been a good thing.

My activities at church were another large part of my life during high school. As I already mentioned, this is where I met Cindy. We became great friends, even though she attended our rival school, Rising Sun High School. She lived directly behind the farm and visiting each other was all we could do whenever we were grounded. We both loved the Beatles, eating Bugles, and could talk for hours. Being in the youth group at church was great and Cindy and I shared that time in our lives. It was a good bunch led by Clarence and Patsy. They opened their house to us, and every season of the year meant something different to do at their house. From cookouts, to sledding, and indoor games in their basement, we were kept busy. The people at the church in North East meant so much to us as they helped us grow and kept us in line. Being a preacher's kid meant many eyes are upon you and at the strangest times; and living in a small town left no place to hide from all those eyes of people who, for the most part, cared about me. Betty Jackson was one that especially kept me in line during my high school years and was always there to talk to if needed. Later, Patsy Payne came into my life during a confusing time in my life as a mentor and great listener and helped me come to terms with many of my spiritual questions. A good talk with a wise woman can do wonders in the middle of confusing times. My Mom was a phone call away. During these years in my life, I would struggle with spiritual things. Doubt can be good as it makes you search to discover what is real. Do not be afraid to question truth as truth will always prevail.

I had a few jobs during high school. For a little while, I worked at Shallcross' in the town of Rising Sun. That is where I learned all about scrapple and still ate it! My longest job in high school was at Calvert Manor Nursing Home. I was the dishwasher. If I think about it, I can still smell the wash room. Later I worked at Chrome Dairy in Chrome, PA. These jobs kept me on the road. Gas in those days was $.35 a gallon. Just think, my friends and I would gather up change, and a couple of dollars gave us plenty of gas to run on!

Church stories as the preacher's kid are always part of my memory. One Sunday while Dad was preaching, our group was sitting together in the back, but not quite in the back row. Dad had warned me often about our group talking during his sermon and he did have a great view of us from the platform. This particular Sunday he suddenly stopped preaching and said, "Donna, come up here and sit with your mother." Now I am certain I had not been talking, but he saw someone else talking. That place got very quiet as I obeyed and came to the FRONT row to sit by Mom. It was a long time before any of the youth talked during his sermon again. I do not remember being real upset. I guess that was just the life of the preacher's kid! I do remember many of Dad's sermons to this day. One that stands out is "Little Foxes Spoil the Vine" from a verse in Song of Solomon. It is so true that the little things are often what trip us in our lives. Other sermons such as "Keep the Jelly on the Bottom Shelf", which referred to keeping the important things reachable, helped me to focus on priorities. There was also the time he got a few words backwards and said, "Moses, take off your feet you are standing on holy ground", and the snickers rumbled around the room. Dad was also a master at memorizing poetry that he often used in his sermons. These are just a few of my vivid memories.

Now I have told you some stories about my high school years, but other stories, as I promised, will remain only in my distant memory. I do not recommend being wild and reckless in order to learn, but I must admit through the years God has taught me much about his love, mercy, and grace because of where I have been, and He was preparing me for where He wanted to take me. It is a miracle any of us make it to adulthood.

For someone who had spent most of my school years hating it, by the time I was a senior I was loving school. During my senior year, about December, Dad resigned from the church as he had been called to a church in Indiana. Leaving Maryland and NEHS was the last thing I wanted to do in the middle of my senior year. Dad and Mom talked to Nee Nee and Pop Pop and made arrangements for me to stay with them to finish out the year. They had built a nice little place on a corner of the farm property after they sold the farm. They made the spare room my room and welcomed me into their home. They loved me very much. I loved my grandparents dearly, but they were my grandparents. Grandparents usually do not make good disciplinarians, and I still needed plenty of guidance. They tried, but I had many new found freedoms for the rest of the year. Thankfully I did not get into any serious trouble, but about drove my grandparents crazy. I really depended on Rick and Mary Etta Reedy during these months and years following high school, and credit them with helping me to grow up a little as they continued to remind me that wrong actions have consequences. June finally came and I did graduate and moved to Indiana for the summer and gave my grandparents a period of rest.

Indiana was difficult to make home. My family was there and I sure did miss my family, but my friends were in Maryland. I did make some friends at the new church where Dad was pastor, but always wanted to be back in Maryland. There were some good people at that church, but there were some hard times, too. Good or bad, they are one of my circles. Dad went through some tough times as a pastor and working with people over the years. I am thankful those times did not make me bitter toward church or the people involved. Sadly, I learned that Christians can be just as wicked as anyone else.

At the church in Indiana, Dad was having some difficulties with some church members, especially, one man. After one meeting where Dad was really beat up with some awful words, I took it very hard. As a family we had gone to the house that was just across the parking lot, when this particular man came to the back door to continue his barrage of words. By this time in my life, I was seventeen years old and still very much a tomboy. I was so frustrated by what this man had said to my Dad that I stepped between them and punched him in the stomach. Dad was upset with me on the outside and sent me into the house immediately, but I like to think he was laughing on the inside. When this man died many years later of a stomach aneurysm, I felt guilty as if I had been responsible, although I know I was not.

Dad resigned from the church and eventually started a new church in another small town. A little later, the previous church burned to the ground and Dad visited the church property and cried over the destruction, as he had poured years of hard work into that church. I must say that I felt they received their just dues. Lynn and I were working at Kentucky Fried Chicken during this time and were questioned, jokingly, as to whether we had anything to do with the church that burned. Lynn and I did not do it, although after the Kentucky Fried

Chicken also burned to the ground we did look suspicious. We did not burn this place either, as we loved working there with some great managers and all the fried livers and gizzards we could ever eat.

Forgiveness… Something we all must practice. Unchecked anger and unforgiveness leads to bitterness and bitterness only hurts YOU, not the offender. God has forgiven me so what greater reason do I have to forgive those who hurt me. As a result of those difficult years as a preacher's daughter and watching people hurt my Dad, I had the need to learn to forgive others, although they never asked for my forgiveness. Learn to willingly forgive the hurts others cause. Please don't carry unforgiveness as everyone around you will suffer from the consequences. Forgive. Run to it…Give it…Live a life of forgiveness. It is healing to your own soul. Put away anger as anger destroys you and your relationships. Practice self-control and control anger. People will make mistakes, whether accidently or on purpose. Learning to forgive and move on only makes one stronger.

My love for sports continued, and there was nothing better than a backyard game of basketball with Dad or football with a group of friends. In one football game, I tackled a guy who was the quarterback on his high school team and broke his shoulder. Obviously, this did not make his coach very happy. Being young and involved in whatever was happening at the moment, kept me going. I was and still am a people-person and want to be where the action is! This was a major change from that little girl before high school.

Another good thing about being the Pastor's daughter was taking a mission's trip. We, as a family, went to Spanish Wells, Bahamas, and suffered there for Jesus for a month. We flew from Miami in a small airplane. As we waited for the pilot to arrive, someone told us he was "downstairs getting up nerve to fly this thing". This was not very comforting to Mom, and I was nervous, too. Flying was never my favorite thing to do. When the pilot came, he told us not to worry as this little plane was very easy to land in the water if necessary. Again, not very comforting, but it was a great trip. The best crawfish and grouper in the world are found in those beautiful waters, along with the Johnny cake and couch salad that can be found in Spanish Wells. I made many friends in Spanish Wells, who are friends to this day. There are many tales that could be told of my adventures on Spanish Wells. Pam and Cheryl keep in touch on a regular basis and they are one of my circles. I have been back for a visit and the door is always open with a place to stay! It is nice to have dear friends in such a beautiful spot in the world!!

No matter where life takes you, there will always be a special place in your heart for that place you call home. For me that place is Cecil County, Maryland. It is a great place that I have called home most of my life. The rolling hills, farmlands, plentiful trees, four seasons, waterways, luscious grass and great people are enough to call me back. In Maryland, spring is for planting and watching the earth come to life as the flowers and trees begin to bloom. June brings the strawberries, July brings tomatoes, August brings peaches and sweet corn and September brings the apples. Summer is also for lazy days, picnics and time at the beach. Fall is for cool days with evening bonfires, long walks and enjoying the beautiful colors. Winter is for family gatherings at holidays, wonderful snowfalls that blanket the barren land and the smell of cobblers, stews, pies, turkey and chili. The memories are the sweetest of home.

Eventually I did go back to Maryland. As a matter of fact, I moved back and forth a few times trying to get settled. Remember, I am a slow learner, typically learning the hard way, and was very restless as I searched for my spot in this world. I enrolled at Cecil Community College and did okay even though I played more card games and attended more parties than studied. Later, I attended Lancaster Bible College and Liberty University online. This is not the way to complete college. When I would go back to Indiana I would get a job and stay a little while, helping out at Dad's church. My real desire was to be in Maryland.

Once when I came back to Maryland, Michael Owens was on the corner by the store in Zion with Steve Foster as I drove through Zion. Michael had just been honorably discharged from the United States Army in February after serving for three years in Germany. He and Steve had once again picked up on their old habits. They hung out there often and this was my lucky day. He wondered what I was doing and decided to call and ask me out. That was in April, 1971, and Cindy and Steve were about to get married. It ended up that our first date was April 24, 1971, Steve and Cindy's wedding night. What were the chances that our best friends were getting married? Steve and Michael had grown up together since babies.

After the wedding in Zion, Michael picked me up at my grandparent's house and we went to the movies, only after I made him wait as I brushed my teeth and watched him out the bathroom window. My grandmother's house that night smelled of broiled Rock fish as their dear friends, Dot and Ben Sauselein, were coming for dinner. The smell of Rock fish will always remind me of our first date. I knew coming back to Maryland was the right thing! This is when those Barracudas fell in love. Michael took me to his parent's house that evening, told them I followed him home, and asked if he could keep me. As he went upstairs to change his clothes, he told his parents to keep me off the furniture. Michael is always being the comedian.

This was a restless period of my life, as I did not know what I wanted to do. Growing up can be so hard! Michael was in my life and I knew I had found a good man, but it would have been just too easy to let him catch me quickly and I loved playing hard to get. I lived with Rick and Mary Etta Reedy for awhile and then moved to Aunt Kay and Uncle Clarence's house. I worked at Chrome Dairy in Pennsylvania during this time. Later I apologized to my grandparents for the grief I had caused them and being grandparents they had long ago forgiven me. I know I gave Nee Nee a few more gray hairs, only adding to the ones my Dad and Ruthie had already given her. Michael was good for me and soon became my steadying factor!

Now I had a different purpose for being in Maryland, but my family was still so far away in Indiana. I missed my parents, but really missed Lynn and Deneen, too. They were growing up and I was not there to see all the changes. Even though Lynn and I still would have a fight after a few days of being in the same house, we still enjoyed being together and my baby sister was not a baby anymore. If I went to Indiana, Michael would visit. On one visit I even broke up with him, and he left driving on to Denver alone. On his way back East, we got back together again. What a man I had found who put up with my nonsense! When in Maryland, Michael and I spent much time together. I always enjoyed spending time with his family, too! I can never say enough about his family who love me as their own.

We spent many hours with Steve and Cindy. We doubled dated often, spending time at their apartment in Newark, or perhaps going to a drive-in movie. We had some great times hanging out as friends. We knew we were getting old when we all decided that 10:30 PM was getting late. Michael and Steve both had motorcycles and we enjoyed many rides exploring the countryside. Once we took a trip together to Cape May on the motorcycles. If you could see the pictures of that trip, you would say we were hippies!

The day came during one of my trips back to Maryland, and we were heading home one night from a date, that Michael stopped the car after turning onto Trinity Church Road near Zion, and right there he asked me to marry him. Obviously, I said yes! This time I went back to Indiana with an engagement ring and a wedding to plan. That was a big job for Mom, as the wedding was to be in Maryland. Sisters, Lynn and Deneen, sisters-in-law to be, Sharon and Charlotte, and dear friend, Cindy, were all asked to be a part of the big day. Michael chose Steve, brothers-in-law, and two of my cousins, Dennis and Craig. Dennis and Craig were chosen by lottery. Walter Burcham and Dad were to do the ceremony. It was great to have Dad willing to give me away and participate in the ceremony. One more time, I moved back to Maryland and got the apartment in Zion. The apartment was Jim and Ann Renn's house, and right up the street from Steve and Cindy. I also got a job at Sopher's Department Store in Oxford and continued going to school. I worked there until after we were married. Sopher's is where I found my wedding dress. Aunt Kay, Mom and my girls gave me a beautiful bridal shower in Conowingo. I had found my true love. Michael had become my best friend after I had finally allowed him to catch me.

We were married on June 9, 1973, 7:00 PM, at the church in Conowingo where I had spent my early childhood days. Aunt Kay and Uncle Clarence allowed us to use their house to get ready for the wedding as it was right across the road from the church. Dad did walk me down the aisle, looking more nervous in that tuxedo than I had ever seen him before. Michael was waiting for me at the altar in his blue tuxedo with a swirled design. After the ceremony and reception at the church, we came to the apartment to change and leave for our honeymoon while the church bells were ringing at the little church in Zion in celebration of our day. And so began another part of the journey... old circles were joining with new circles as life continues.

Chapter 4

Journey into Marriage

Joys are more joyful and burdens are so much lighter when shared.

Marriage is an incredible journey and one I highly recommend. Marriage requires many things from each person, but the right attitude is most important. The first thing is to take the word divorce out of your vocabulary. Don't get me wrong here...ugly things happen, people can change and you can run out of options. This is the number one reason to head into a marriage only after some serious counsel. Get to know that person and the family, as you marry the family, too! The Bible tells us to love one another. It is a command. You obey a command and the obeying does not depend on how you feel at the moment. Marriage requires commitment and work. Some days we did not feel like we wanted to love each other, but on June 9th we made a commitment to love for a lifetime! Knowing myself, I knew I must beware of criticism (1 Cor. 13), beware of thinking too highly of myself (Romans 12:2-4) and remember I am never alone (Zephaniah 3:17). We also had some great examples as Michael's parents were married 59 years before his Dad passed away and my parents just past 60 years. Most young people think they have regrets...if only I had done_____ or married _____. But I know God's hand of control was and is on our lives. I realize there were other choices I could have made, and He gives us the ability to choose, but how thankful I am to look back and see his hand of guidance through all our years. The "what ifs" in life no longer matter as we do not get to go back and start again. Don't miss the life in front of you wondering what might have been.

Our honeymoon has many special memories. First of all, Steve and Cindy took us to the airport, and Michael had reserved a hotel room for our first night. They helped us carry everything to the room and we said our goodbyes. The room had a bottle of champagne, and I remember the top shooting off as Michael opened it. That was fun, but we both considered the taste terrible. We planned on that being our last taste, too! Jumping quickly to the next day...We went to the airport and soon boarded a plane for Denver. Michael had planned a two week adventure in the Denver area. As we boarded the plane, we were easily spotted, as newlyweds often are, and introduced to the Captain in the cockpit. Michael's Uncle Pete (Olin Grubb), who was also a United Airlines pilot and has an incredible life story well worth reading, set up the meeting. Once in flight on the United Airline plane, an announcement came over the intercom. They welcomed us as newlyweds, everyone applauded, and we were given a small cake and another bottle of champagne exactly like the last one! When we arrived in Denver, Michael left me sitting with the entire luggage, the cake and that bottle of champagne, as he went to rent a car. The comments from people included "Oh, he left you already?" We had a great time traveling into the mountains enjoying the snow in June, eating sourdough pancakes at the ranch in Jackson Hole, watching whitecaps on the swimming pool in Cheyenne, visiting Yellowstone National Park complete with the spewing of Old Faithful, a lone moose in a field and a Grizzly bear beside the road. It was a very special trip. On the way home, we flew to Indiana to visit my parents for a couple of days. Now it was time for settling in to being married and living our daily lives.

This man I married, Michael Alan Owens, is so consistent... Mr. Organization! And best of all he loves me completely and unconditionally. I was and still am completely secure in our relationship. I knew he was with me for the long haul. Michael is not a quitter and his commitment is for life. He was, and is, my compass through my still growing up process. Yes, and I call him Michael though others may call him Mike. His Mom has always referred to him as Michael, and I kept up the tradition.

We had many ups and downs as the years went by. Those times have created the marriage we have today. Our love is strong and the bonds are permanent. I don't think our sons ever worried that one of us would leave. We really did mean "till death do us part". Now a couple of times over the years we almost caused one another's early death. I guess I should insert here the "best" fight we ever had. I must jump way ahead in time for this story as we were in our house on McCauley Road. The boys were young, but old enough to remember. It had been an unusually busy day for both of us, and we were ready to quit for the day. But there was one more job to be done. Mrs. Daly had sent some apples down and they were ready to be applesauce. I began the process of cooking, straining and preparing the sauce for the freezer. Frozen applesauce is one of my favorite foods. The next events are blurred. A bag broke, I got angry (hard to imagine), Michael walked in the kitchen, made a comment, and applesauce began to fly. We BOTH threw applesauce everywhere. Finally, as we looked around at the mess we had created, even on the ceiling, we sat down and laughed until we cried. The clean up was a long process and because of the acid in the apples we needed to paint the kitchen a few days later! This obviously was not our only fight, but a memorable one. Once again the bumps along the way caused growth and we have grown together. Remember, that is a choice-you can grow together or you can grow apart. Perhaps I should add that we grew up together in this wild ride called marriage.

Now back to the order of things! Michael and I enjoyed living in our apartment. We had a living room and very small kitchen downstairs and two bedrooms and a bathroom upstairs. It was a large house and the other half was an apartment also. With our wedding gifts, money and hand-me-downs we were able to nicely furnish the place. Oh, we had so much to learnJ. First of all, I was not a cook. I had never stayed still long enough to learn to cook, but I had great teachers in Mom and my grandmothers and I finally realized cooking was a necessity. I don't remember those first meals, I wonder if Michael does? Thankfully, there were no smoke alarms.

Here we were living back in Zion, the little village I had grown up in so many years ago, and Michael had lived all his life other than Army years. Michael was now working at Carson's Garage in Rising Sun. Before we were married, he had worked at the garage in Zion with his Dad. So we were surrounded by people that knew us very well, yet loved us. We knew Julia Touchton, who had known us from babies, and lived next door, spied on us and knew our every move. Michael's parents lived three houses up, but they were never ones to interfere in our lives unless we asked. If we asked, they would do anything for us. I must say now that I have the best in-laws ever. His Dad was born and raised in Cecil County and his Mom was born in Battle Creek, Nebraska, and their combined life experiences and wisdom benefited us greatly through the years.

At the beginning of our marriage, I was still working at Sopher's in Oxford, going to college and began substitute teaching. Michael and I both liked our apartment. We had a pet at the apartment – a parakeet named Heathcliff. Crazy thing was messy, throwing seeds everywhere. He died while we were away one time. Living there was a good beginning, but it was time to move on.

From Zion we moved to the Port Deposit, Maryland area. Being tired of paying rent and wanting to put our money into a house, we began to look. Now we weren't exactly rich, so the shopping for a house was narrow. By this time in our lives we had settled into church in that area, so looking in the Port direction made sense. Michael found a mobile home in a nice park on Rt. 276. The price was right, but the place was very dirty, mostly from smoke. We spent several days cleaning before we could move in.

About that time we were given a kitten that someone found under a car in McDonalds parking lot. We named him Mac. Mac settled in for many months. One day Mac disappeared and was gone for months. Once, while Michael was working night shift, that cat followed him in the door and walked over to where his dish once was as if he had never left. I could hardly believe my eyes. He had been injured, but was now healed with part of a leg and his tail missing. Someone surely took care of him after such an injury. Mac moved with us to Hilltop and eventually to McCauley Road before meeting his demise. Sometime later another cat entered our lives and stayed around for 20 years!

During these few years in the park, Michael changed jobs and began working at Monsanto in Havre de Grace, Maryland. He had a good job with promise until they had problems with the plastic bottles that bottled Coke. So the plant closing took him to his most difficult job at P & R Railcar in Elkton, Maryland. He worked very hard and it was dirty work, yet he did not complain. I had been asked to work with the youth at our church and continued working on college classes in class and online. One of my many mistakes was not to finish college before marriage…just a note of advice to anyone listening. We were busy and too often going in different directions. My focus too often was on me and not us. It is easy to become selfish in relationships. In our marriage it needed to be more "us", instead of "me".

We again had another circle of friends forming. Many of them are still on the fringes of my life today. Cultivate friendships along your journey even if they are only for a brief moment in time. Being vulnerable to others is risky, but friends are worth the risk. As with many friendships, some fade away as our circumstances change, while others endure the test of time. I am thankful for so many friendships that last over time. People like Candy, Andrea (Andy), Marlene, Debbie and Donna entered my circle with friendships that are treasured. Donna was younger and settled into our family as one of our own children. Old friends are people with whom we can pick up wherever we left off when we see one another. Such friendships are to be cherished and nourished. I am especially thankful for the ones that have become lifelong friends.

It was in the spring of 1976 that I finally realized it was time to work on growing up. My relationship with God became more personal as I saw the importance of a personal quiet time with God. I had grown up with the Bible, but suddenly Scripture became more real to me. I was beginning to understand my constant need for God. My spiritual journey began as a child, yet changed drastically during this time. I will always go back to this time as a young adult knowing my personal relationship with God was solidified. Some people are just slow maturing spiritually, physically and mentally. The growing still is not complete, as only death should end our growing, but at least the process had begun. Working with the teenagers helped to keep me focused. Someone was always watching. As I was beginning to understand the need to be a positive role model, my life became more focused. The youth kept me busy with all their activities and another change was coming.

By now it is August, 1976. Michael and I had talked about having children, but that wasn't happening just yet. Once again, God knew I was far from ready to be a mom. One day during the month I received a phone call from Uncle Ben. He asked what I was doing and if I would be interested in a job at Hilltop Ranch, Colora, Maryland. Church and substituting were keeping me busy enough, but I was interested. I went for an interview and met Jim Roberts, an encounter that really changed our lives! Being hired that day, I had no idea the variety of experiences I was about to delve into. The Morning Cheer family and many staff from all over the country entered my life. We influenced many over the years at Hilltop and in turn were influenced by so many. This job was to be quite a ride and a great circle.

I began working in the office...my experience being what I had learned working part-time in the church office. But this job was much more than an office job. Summer camp had ended and rental groups were arriving every weekend and sometimes through the week. As the summer staff went home or back to college, one of my jobs was to call from the list of local high school students and fill the kitchen and dining room staff needs for the weekends. The groups that arrived through the week were much more difficult to staff. My job description had listed many responsibilities and ended with a line that said, "And any other duties deemed necessary." So the fun began. During my years at Hilltop not only did I work in the office, but served tables, helped cook, learn to run games and activities, and even learned to lifeguard. Jim Roberts was a great boss. He taught me so much especially about servant/leadership. His choice in a wife was a great choice also as Sharon was a dear friend. Our experiences at Hilltop created friendships that have lasted over time. We even attended some college classes together at Lancaster Bible College. Jim enjoyed introducing me to new and wild things. Becoming a lifeguard was crazy. Jim taught the class and among the students was my cousin, Ronnie. Growing up we called Ronnie, "Lumpy" for a reason. He is a big guy. For my final test in the class, I was required to go into the pool and "rescue" someone who was drowning. Now the "drowning" victim had no boundaries. Ronnie was chosen to be the one I would rescue. First he went to the bottom of the pool at the deepest part, and he just laid there. When I finally got him off the bottom of the pool he fought me all the way to the side. I was exhausted, but had just earned my lifesaver card. So when groups would use the pool, I was called on often. Some days it was down the hill to lifeguard, then up the hill to wait on tables, only to return to the office to finish the work there. Sometimes I worked in the snack shop plus helped make hundreds of donuts or pizzas for arriving groups when the need arose. Oh, the stories I could tell of Hilltop. It was far from a boring office job. Jim also taught me to rock climb and rappel. My first rappelling experience was off the roof of the gym, then on to climb and rappel the King and Queen seat in Harford County multiple times. Climbing and repelling at 100+ feet taught me many lessons on trust, finishing the task and reaching the goal. These lessons were both physical and spiritual. In the winter we sledded on the hill and used the great toboggan run. Jim introduced us to snow skiing and we spent many winter days on the slopes in Pennsylvania. One summer he sent me on a canoe trip up the Susquehanna River once with a group of campers in our 34' canoe and Jim Yearsley! Jim Roberts also loved to plan all-nighters and we would all get involved. Every time by about 4 am, we all declared we would never do this again...but we did. Each season brought people to Hilltop...from summer camp to retreats. My experiences at Hilltop were varied. My self-confidence grew.

The summer of 1977 brought more change to my life. One day while working in the office, I received a phone call from Ruthie. Pop Pop Criswell had been taken to the hospital in Havre de Grace. I was allowed to leave immediately and headed there. By the time I reached the hospital, he was in a coma and being transferred to University Hospital in Baltimore. Dad flew in first and soon Mom, Lynn and Deneen were on their way from Indiana. Pop Pop lived two more weeks. He never regained consciousness. His death had a large impact on my life. Sometimes you just think people will always be there. Say "I love you" often.

By the summer of 1978, Hilltop had hired Michael as their maintenance man and we moved to a house on the property at Hilltop. We enjoyed this house and living at camp. It was a two-story house that included two bedrooms and a bath upstairs and a kitchen, dining room, living room, family room and bath downstairs. The living room had a cozy fireplace with a large window that overlooked the fields and hills. Ruthie said "on a clear day you can see forever" out that window and thought that line would make a great song. We both worked there until the late winter/spring of 1982. During the summer camp and winter retreats, we ate our meals in the dining hall on the hill with the other staff. It was a very busy time for us, but once again some years I would not trade. Deneen came and spent some time with us at Hilltop and that was very special. It was a time of getting to know my little sister as a teenager. Many great memories were at Hilltop…the best being the birth of our firstborn. You should try serving tables with a baby on your back. Jim and Sharon Roberts had twins so they each had a baby on their back. Everything changed when Darrell was born and he spent his first year at Hilltop. More on his birth later! I will include the story which I wrote in 1981 after Darrell was born.

Daily living was not exactly normal at camp, but our home was a good hideaway from the action at the top of the hill. My favorite TV show was M.A.S.H. 4077th and I loved to cuddle with Michael and Mac when we had some down time. Darrell's arrival would add a new and exciting dimension to this inner circle.

Hilltop, being a part of Morning Cheer, came into some financial problems. As staff at Hilltop, we did all we could to help, but in 1982 Michael said find us a place to live and we moved. It was time for more lessons on what is important. Our lives had already changed greatly when in December of 1980, Darrell was born. Now, fourteen months later, we were moving and with no job. As a family we would make it.

Chapter 5

Journey with Children

Remembering...

I will never forget a very special time in our lives that resulted in the birth of our firstborn son, Darrell Criswell Owens. We really wanted a baby. We began going to the Quarryville Family Health Center in early 1980. There we met Dr. Phyllis Oblander. After many tests and one more blood test, one Wednesday morning in June as a Christian school was leaving Hilltop, I called the office to find out the results of the blood test. The response, "The test is positive." Not being sure I really believed it I sat at my desk for a moment then began to cry. Ben was in his office next to mine as I ran out saying something about a baby!

Michael was at the top of the stairs to the lobby. That moment in our lives will always be special. Jim was in the dish room as we entered and told him. He had a pleased yet puzzling look on his face. Later we understood why as Sharon had just found out the same news.

After talking to Dr. Oblander to really confirm the news, we called my family in Indiana. Later that evening we stood in the kitchen in Zion telling Michael's Mom and Dad the news. I remember telling Cindy about the baby that late spring as she was standing in her garden quite pregnant with Ryan.

Even the visits to the doctor were fun. We asked so many questions. Every strange pain or feeling was questioned. Dr. O probably laughed each time we left the office.

It was so fun being pregnant the same time as Sharon. We compared notes all the time. The Riopan industry increased for several months. I will always remember hearing the heartbeat and feeling life for the first time. January 6th was to be the due date and seemed soooo far away. My size is another story. There is a picture of Sharon and me sitting in a swing at the Robert Fulton Inn in December. It really shows the whole story (at least Sharon was carrying two).

Christmas day came and went and I was getting restless. On Saturday, December 27th I began having strange pains. We called Dr. O and she wanted to see me. After the office exam she said things were getting started, but that we had plenty of time. She suggested Michael get something to eat as the night could be long. We head for McDonalds, but as we passed the Country Kitchen we saw a familiar car. Michael's parents were a little surprised to see us. Michael ate a meal and I drank a Sprite. Soon we left for Lancaster General Hospital. Excitement plus fear of the unknown were taking over. We had it all so well planned. After all we had taken the classes and I was ready to begin my "breathing" with my "coach" by my side.

We may have been in the labor room two hours when it was decided this baby wanted to wait awhile. Because I was having blood pressure problems, it was decided that I should stay. I thought nine months was long; three days is like forever. The morning of December 30th started very early. My water broke by 5:00 am. With Dr. Oblander on her way in, I called Michael saying "Hurry, I need you!"

Back to the labor room it was for me. Dr. Oblander came in and sat on the side of my bed. Before she left us so she could prepare for the day's events, she prayed a prayer I will always remember. Together we acknowledged God's total control of our lives. I did not know how much I would need that assurance during the next few hours. Those hours in the labor room went on and on. There was a woman screaming a few rooms down. That was real encouraging.

Michael was super. He pushed on my back during contractions (as that was what I wanted) until he was sore and tired. By 4:00 pm the contractions were 45 seconds apart but there was no progress. This baby had a mind of his own and could not be convinced to enter this world. I was so tired that I was falling asleep between contractions.

You see this son started his entrance into this world pulling his Mom's chain and has succeeded to do it quite well since. He had flipped around so much that the cord was now wrapped around his neck several times. The decision was made that a C-section was necessary and crucial to the baby's life. Dr. Oblander left Michael and me to ourselves for a few moments to try to adjust to the idea. At that point things went quickly. As I was ready to enter the operating room, Dr. Oblander reminded me of our prayer that morning. God was in control. Even though I was disappointed, I was ready to do whatever necessary to get this baby here.

The anesthetist asked me my weight, I motioned him closer and whispered the answer and soon I was out. (That answer is too much to write.)

The next thing I remembered was Dr. Oblander telling me, "Darrell is here and he's fine". He was born at 4:50 pm and weighed 8 lbs. 2 ounces. Michael was in the nursery and holding him. As soon as I left recovery I was taken straight to the nursery and he was brought to me.

My emotions took over as I finally held our beautiful baby boy in my arms. Our lives had just changed (little did I know how much) forever.

Back in the room we began to make our phone calls. Mom was first. We both cried. I always knew how special Mom was to me, but for the first time I understood what I was to her. I knew she loved me, but that day I knew how much! Granddaddy and Grandmom arrived soon to hold their new grandson.

Those days in the hospital were special in spite of being so sore. (Walk, walk, and walk) Michael was there for many feeding times and we would sit in bed and count fingers and toes on our new son. Quickly we realized how much Darrell looks like his Daddy. Slowly we began to realize how much he acts like his Mommy. Perhaps the latter will change.

Darrell, what was life like without you? You've kept us awake, made us laugh and cry (tears of happiness), kept us busy taking care of you, and kept us young and made us old at the same time. Most of all, you keep us examining ourselves because God has entrusted us with you and that's a big responsibility.

I sure do love being called Mom. Lord,
make me worthy of such a calling.
I love you, Darrell!

For Darrell: Psalms 32:8 NKJV "I will instruct you and teach you in the way you should go; I will guide you with my eye."

Mom came to Maryland to help after Darrell came home. Dad showed up too! Mom had a wonderful way of taking care of the household chores and cooking great meals so I could focus on Darrell. Ruthie let us borrow the family cradle to use downstairs. Darrell was the fourth generation to sleep in that cradle. Michael's parents came over often, too. Granddaddy built the toy box we still use today. This was such a crazy time of our lives working at camp and learning to be Mom and Dad. Now that I was a Mom, I realized I knew nothing about motherhood and nursing does not come naturally. I almost gave up on the latter. My Mom and Mother-in-law were priceless assets and Darrell actually grew.

We moved that winter/spring of 1982 into a very small 10' X 50' trailer that we found to rent. Even in the Christian world, things are not always perfect. This was a very difficult time in our lives. Circumstance caused us to move from Hilltop and when Michael decided it was time, the move was fast. Boxing up most of our belongings, except for the essentials because of the lack of space, we scattered those boxes and extras from the Owens' to Ruthie's and to Nee Nee's. Michael had no job or insurance. Darrell was 14 months old and very busy. Many emotions flowed that day and now the hunt was on for a house that we could afford to buy. Darrell also ended up very sick with an upper respiratory infection and landed in the hospital for a few days. We took turns staying with him day and night with Grandmom in the mix. Also, during this time Michael found a job and began working for Aberdeen Proving Ground, but the job, for the moment, was temporary.

Another change during the year of 1981 was with Nee Nee. She had met and started spending time with Ralph Townsend, affectionately known as Townie. They were married in the spring of 1981 and Townie became a part of our lives for many years. They provided great companionship for each other and Townie loved us all just as his own.

Back to the house...Now how were we to buy a house on a temporary job after having worked in a ministry for the past several years on a meager salary? Somehow this seemed like a tall order for God to fill. But...we had seen Him faithful to meet our needs so many times before.

There was a man at our church, Duke Snyder, who was a real estate agent and a friend. He had an old house on his hands that he wasn't sure how he was going to sell. He told us about this little house on McCauley Road that needed some tender loving care. He said it has a stream running beside it that was just calling out for a family to have a picnic. When we saw that place and took the tour, we certainly had to look with different eyes to view its potential. The work seemed overwhelming and we needed someone to give us a mortgage. It was fall of 1982. The first step with the mortgage company that even considered us was to write a letter about why we wanted this house. They did not like the word temporary in front of Michael's job either. We got the mortgage! The mortgage rate was crazy (15 7/8%), but the price for the house was right, so it worked for now. Next, we were in the process of moving again.

Packing the few things we had moved into the trailer was a pretty simple task. We really did just live on necessities. Darrell was quite the helper. He had a few prized possessions of his own, one being his "Choo Choo". That little train ran the rail of his crib, but when it stopped if he wasn't asleep, we had to start all over again. This move was an adventure for us all.

On moving week as we were packing and loading things into the car, and Darrell carried the picture of Mom and Dad (Granny and Pop) across the living room to the door. Just as he opened the door Granny and Pop came walking up the sidewalk. Darrell had a very puzzled look on his face as if they had just walked out of that picture. Actually, they surprised us all. They proved to be a big help in cleaning the house so we could move in. One major job on the day of settlement was stripping all the floors of the old carpet that covered them. As we began pulling up layers of carpet in the living room, we discovered hardwood flooring. It was in rough shape. Michael's Dad, Granddaddy, took it upon himself to hand sand and polyurethane the floor. As with every piece of antique furniture or project he took on, he did the job with excellence. My Dad, Pop, stayed busy removing staples and unwanted nails from the walls and floors and making any repairs needed. Michael's Mom, Grandmom, scrubbed that old kitchen and cupboards until spotless. My Mom, Granny, washed windows until they sparkled, except for the one she broke. With all the help, we were able to move in and Michael began one room at a time to upgrade. One major project he accomplished over time was the deck in the back. That area has become my gardens and is enjoyed throughout the year. It didn't take Darrell long to learn to climb the winding stairs to the second floor. He was always reminded to use the wide part. Over the years these stairs have been the back drop for many pictures, especially on my cherished Christmas mornings.

Moving into this old house was fun. We gathered all the boxes that were scattered in various basements. We had labeled them well as to the contents, but opening them and going through our stuff was like Christmas. Of course, if we lived without this stuff for over a year, did we really need it? Yes, we did! There were pictures, knick knacks, and all the extras that make a house a home. With those winding stairs so many things would not fit and Michael had to take out the entire window and frame in the hall and move things in through that window after hoisting them on the back roof. Those dressers and beds were there to stay!

This old house has always given us projects, and Michael and I have spent many hours upgrading. Some of our dreams and plans with this old house have not happened, but somehow moving has just never seemed an option. This place is full of cherished memories providing our own little escape from the world, the solitude we needed to be a family, and a place to enjoy backyard times with friends and family. Down by the stream has provided many hours of tranquility. The large rock is a part of so many family pictures. The rock was the jumping off point for the boys using a rope swing from the tree. When a storm one year took out that old tree, I knew we needed to plant another one quickly so someday my grandchildren would be able to swing off that rock. Later, we were able to put in a swimming pool that brought hours of enjoyment for us all as a family and with friends. Michael spent hours building the decking and we worked on the landscaping together. Later, we would remodel the back dining room that allowed room for an Amish made 10 foot table to meet the needs of our growing family. With the surrounding woods, farms, pond, stream and great neighbors, it has been the perfect place to raise a family.

Let me stop here to talk about possessions. Beware of ownership. Every possession has the ability to own you, whether you are rich or poor. Things are a time stealer. They take you away from the more important part of life...PEOPLE. Keep THINGS in perspective. Bigger and better had been a goal when we purchased this old house, but as time went on, this old home was too precious to sell. Today we are freer because of our decision to stay in this house. Seek counsel on decisions and be wise. You are not the sum of what you own.

Over the years, we have gathered some things and some of those have family value. In a little book I have written a list of those collected items and a brief history of where they came from. Our sons will need to decide who gets what, with the exception of the china cabinet that belongs to Alisha and this old table, whose story I will include, has been claimed by Jared. I could be like Mom Mom Clark and start having the family put their name on the bottom of things they would like to have. The point is things can hold special meaning, but they can never replace the people. Things are temporary, but people are forever. The following is a story written to us by Grandmom (Kathleen Owens) for Christmas 1988. Enjoy it and treasure it.

CHRISTMAS 1988

Dear Mike & Donna:

I have tried to remember when I first became a table, but I guess that must have been so long time ago that my memory fails me. My first dim memory is of a remote place in England. It was with pride that the first family showed me off in their home. My memory does not recall how long I served that family but then I remember hearing discussions of a wonderful place far away that was called America. One day the family excitedly packed everything (I was afraid I would be left behind) and moved slowly to a place they called a wharf. I was excited about being taken with them, but a little of the thrill was gone when I was packed in a dark place in a little ship. It took weeks of tossing up and down on a place they called the ocean until we reached another wharf in a new country.

The family was excited about being in a new country. I was moved from one place to another and cannot clearly recall all the places I was used. One Lady was a seamstress and I was really used during the stay with her. She used me to cut out all the clothes she made for other people and then she would iron those same clothes on me. I really didn't like that part of my life.

I was used by many people of this same family – one generation and then the next until I was given to Ida and Richard Owens who lived on a farm. Would you believe they had eight children, you know I had an important part in the daily lives there. They often had extra men helping in the fields, so once again I was called into service when they fed the help. Eventually all the six boys and two girls were married or left home to find their own lives.

I was lucky and was taken to the home of the youngest son of that family. I was in the home of Avery Owens for many years. There were two sons, Alfred and Richard. You wouldn't believe the work they did on me. They would cover me with paper and used me for much of the work involved in butchering pigs and beef. I began to wonder how many more types of work could be done on my top. I did like the idea that they used me for the kitchen table and all meals were served on me. After many years in that house the lady of the house, Ethel, decided she wanted to go "modern" and that left me without a job to do.

It was at this time I was given to Alfred and Kitty Owens who lived just down the road in a little place called Zion. Alfred was told that it could be used or stored away, but that it was not be sold or given away outside of the family. That family had one son and two daughters (Michael, Sharon and Charlotte) and I was placed in the living room after a refreshing refinishing job, where I was used to hold a lamp and important family pictures. Quite an easy life compared to some of the jobs I have held in the past.

Several years passed and once again I was caught up in a moving experience. This time it was back up the road to the farm of Avery Owens. (Ethel had died in the meantime.) Space was limited in the living room, so I was placed in the basement where I held the TV and games used by the grandchildren of Alfred and Kitty. (Shane, Christopher Miller; Jinelle, Jacqueline Alexander; Amy Graustein; Darrell and Jared Owens)

Now, at this time – December 1988, I once again am moving into a new home – your home!! I have had a good refinishing job by Alfred and know that I am going to enjoy a renewed spirit of love and care in your home as I serve your family.

THE OWENS' TABLE

(Since that day I have served as the kitchen table for Michael, Donna, Darrell and Jared Owens.)

The Daly's, Ways and Thomas', as our neighbors, had much influence and provided many jobs for the boys over the years. This is the only house the boys knew during their growing up years. Leaving this old house is not even thinkable for now. Remember, this house was to be a stepping stone to something bigger and better. Now these walls share the stories of our lives as a family. The door from the kitchen to the basement shows the years of growth for Darrell, Jared, Dustin, and now the grandsons and includes the dates. These walls will fall someday, but my heart securely holds these stories that I treasure.

Oh yes, boys! Now I need to back up a few years again. Life with another child! Our inner circle was growing. Baby number two was on the way and the following is the story I wrote after his birth. We still had no health insurance and soon learned that you can put your medical expenses of having a baby on a credit card. This is not the recommended route to take, but it worked.

Remember another even so similar, yet so different.

It was May 1983. Some changes were occurring in me that reminded me of another spring. A visit to the doctor, blood test...a positive reading. The excitement is just as great for number two.

I called Michael at Aberdeen and later we shared the news with our families. Another winter baby was coming. Could this one be a girl?

Wow did I ever start showing quickly. As I grew we planned and organized for another baby. Ha-ha this time we were pros! It was exciting sharing it all with Darrell. He enjoyed talking to the baby and hoping it was going to be a brother. We picked names for a boy or girl. The months passed and things went well. Darrell went on the doctor visits with us and we all heard the heartbeat. Somehow carrying a life is so special!

Because Darrell had ended up a C-section, we planned for this one to be a C-section, too, as it was typical in those days. Dr. Murphy gave us a span of two weeks in which to choose the date. January 30th fell in that time period. Since Darrell was December 30th we thought in our old age it would be easy to remember January 30th. So it was set.

I was to be at the hospital by six o'clock on the morning of the 30th. The night before we took Darrell to Grandmom and Granddaddy's to stay until we came home. He was so excited and was praying for his new brother. It was settled in his mind. Michael had never said either way, but I had hoped for a girl. When you get to the point of giving birth all you ask for is a healthy baby.

I was prepped and things were ready to roll. Michael was to be with me and I would be awake for the birth. Michael even had his own personal nurse for the event. Fathers just can't be trusted in delivery!

Wow what an experience! Michael said later that someone should have prepared him for the sucking sound as they pulled out our baby BOY! It was 8:15 am. Such joy we felt at that beautiful sight. Jared Michael Owens was here! Dr. Murphy announced it is a boy and soon I would be holding him. Michael kissed me and in an instant the atmosphere in that room changed! You see this little guy was not to be out done by his big brother. Jared Michael had stopped breathing. He was rushed to a corner of the room that held much equipment and all attention was on HIM! We were so scared and for several minutes there were no answers to our questions.

Finally after what seemed an eternity, Dr. Murphy came back to us. He was breathing, but must go to the neo-natal unit. We never got to hold him! It was such an emotional roller coaster for us.

As they finished with me, Michael went with Jared. Soon I was wheeled to the unit to see Jared through a window. Because I had to lie flat on my back for 24 hours, I could not be with Jared. The nurses were great as they came constantly with updated reports. It was such a comfort to know Michael was with him and brought back reports.

Late afternoon it began to snow. Michael was exhausted and so was I. Also Michael had a long drive home and plus he wanted to see Darrell and tell him about his new brother. When he left I lay there alone and overwhelmed with the day's events. Jared was stable for now.

We had made our phone calls and it was time to rest. It was so hard not seeing Jared or having Michael there to report. Thinking because of the snow, that the night would be long, I was certainly surprised to see my in-laws walk into my room. I immediately sent them to see Jared and bring back a report. And I will repeat that Mom and Dad O. have always been there when we needed them!

Twenty-four hours brought many changes. I was up and holding Jared. Soon Darrell would arrive for his first visit with brother! What a fun time at the hospital. All the tests on Jared were okay and he and I would be home soon.

Two Sons — what a wonderful blessing God has
given us. Thank you Lord for Jared!

I love you, Jared!

_For Jared: Psalm 143:10 NKJV "Teach me to do your will;
for you are my God; your spirit is good; lead me in the land of
uprightness."_

Mom came once again to help. This time she had all the household
chores, plus Darrell to keep up with. Granny spent lots of time with
Darrell. Over the years, every time Granny and Pop came for a visit,
she and Darrell would have a water fight. You can never trust Darrell
with a hose! Darrell was certainly a proud big brother, but I think he
was a little impatient waiting for his brother to be big enough to play.
That time came soon enough. Living in the country, they had only
each other most of the time. I am grateful that they became such good
friends!

I enjoyed being a stay- at- home Mom! With the two boys time
moved quickly looking back, but the day- to-day could be tedious.
Remember how much I have complained about change? Over all the
change I have mentioned I had no control. There is a change I can and
do often control and that is my furniture. Michael often jokes that one
day you will find me in a support group..."Hi, my name is Donna and
I love to move furniture." Michael says if he ever loses his eyesight,
either I quit moving stuff or he gets hurt. Rearranging a room energizes
me. The room feels new, bright and clean. There is always a reason to
rearrange furniture. My desire is to never become a controller of my
family or friends. Their lives, decisions both good and bad, are their
own to make. I pray for them daily and trust God with their lives.
Meanwhile, just let me move furniture!

How I love having boys! Now, I have been ganged up on quite
often by three guys in the house and would not trade it for anything.
Trivial facts have become such an Owens' trademark. Michael's sense of

humor is so contagious and the boys learned quickly. Anyone reading this and thinking Michael is a quiet man has never gotten to know him very well. He chooses his words carefully and demonstrates his wisdom. Some of his jokes are so old, yet always bring a smile or at least a roll of the eyes. An example of an old joke is the one about the fruit peddler who cantaloupe. Certain family members have grown to count on this joke if we are eating cantaloupe. Michael is so much like his father and the blood line runs deep as Jared follows their footsteps. Michael has an often dry sense of humor, a love of little known facts, and can say words such as "palt and sepper" or "coff of cuppy" and on and on as quickly as if it is normal. Another famous line of Michael's is "I saw that in a movie once." The amount of times and the unusual places this line occurs cannot be counted. Strange circumstances often bring out the line. Only this morning as we were awaken to the sounds of many crows Michael and said we were surrounded by Indians, as he saw it in a movie once. His humor keeps us going on even the worst days. The boys affectionately call Dad, "cold water" and rightly so. He can slow down the processes that seem to pour out of the boys and I that are notorious in the Criswell bloodline. The Criswell blood comes with great comebacks. The combination of Owens/Criswell creates optimistic, happy people. The Owens one- liners are renowned, running from Alfred down through his grandsons. Something else I realized recently that runs through the Owens men, is a little smirk that seems to cross their face in so many pictures. Michael's Dad and his Uncle Richard have that smirk in so many photographs and so do our guys! It is fun to watch the sometimes not so subtle effects of bloodlines in the blending families.

Proverbs 17:22 NKJV "A merry heart does good like a medicine."

Children are all so different. We believe each of us has the physical, spiritual, mental and social needs that should be met. Teaching them about God and that Jesus loves them so much that he was willing to die for them was important to us. Darrell, as a little boy sitting with me one day on the front porch swing, wanted Jesus to come and be a part of his life. Jared, as a little boy, on one of our trips to Indiana, told his Pop after church that he wanted Jesus to come and live in his heart and he gave his life to God. Both sons had tender hearts and wanted to live for God. We tried to help them grow in all areas and to realize that it is the relationship with God that is the most important. God always finishes His own work. Life will have hard times along with the good, but an active personal relationship with God will carry you through both.

Darrell can always push my buttons verbally and Jared can do the same with a non-verbal action. The younger is wise to learn from the older. Both sons have the quick comebacks that come with creative minds. Their creativity often had made us laugh. Darrell is creative in getting in and, often, out of trouble. One time he was waiting for his Dad to come to his room for a talk and he knew a spanking was on the way. As he waited, his creative mind caused him to grab a couple of Golden books and place them as a protective barrier in his underwear. Dad noticed. Jared was more cautious as he learned the aggressive ways of his brother brought much swifter discipline. Jared implemented his father's favorite saying, "Hide and Watch" extremely well. Both boys were talented with their hands and as children learned to construct forts, dams, and tree houses. As teenagers, they learned a variety of skills working around home and on the farms. Jared built a loft bed for his small room to use his space wisely. With Dad's help they learned their way around a car engine, too. They both inherited a temper as they had no chance with us as parents. Self control is an attribute we all must continue to work on.

As Mom, I subconsciously and, sometimes, consciously wanted perfect boys. Now the first problem with that is, they have imperfect parents. Pride can and does get in the way of good parenting sense. I look back and realize they were just being kids. They can and will embarrass you, so get used to it. Darrell is our outgoing, get it done, adrenaline junkie son most of the time. Jared is our kind, sensitive, think about it son, most of the time. Both personalities come with big hearts and are fun, yet they will yield different reactions. I learned the traits I enjoyed in one or the other were part of their personality, and the traits I may have wanted in them were not always possible. Keeping myself under control (not always easy) I learned to appreciate them as individuals, striving to help them develop Godly traits that would make them strong men. I can honestly say I love them both for who they are! What pleasure I have in watching them as men. My sons make me smile.

We made many trips to Indiana over the years. Now we could also watch the strong Criswell actions coming through after Darrell was born. It was more complicated after Darrell was born to make the trip to Indiana or any trip for that matter. Why do such little things need so much stuff! His first trip was in March 1981. He did well until the last two hours and decided to cry the rest of the way. Then we added the second son to the mix. I remember that first trip with two as we had to pack diapers around their car seats. We would travel to Indiana every other Christmas. Nee Nee would always have Christmas packages to send. There were two for every person including the bows. Packing the car always meant a fight between Michael and me, but we managed to get everything in for each trip. The trips, other than Christmas, did mean a little less stuff! One trip, Darrell and I went with Nee and Townie to Indiana. While we were there, Darrell got very sick. The day we were to depart came and Nee and Townie decided they needed to get home as the yard must be mowed. Darrell was too sick to travel so they left us behind. About a week later, we hitched a ride with a missionary traveling through Mom and Dad's area. He owned a VW Beetle. I held Darrell in my arms never leaving the car for eight hours straight to Fredrick, Maryland, where Michael met us and took us home. I was never so glad to be home! Over the years there were weddings for Dennis and Lynn and then later Jim and Deneen. Each trip, Granny and Pop always made it special for their grandsons. I will never forget the first time we let Darrell stay out there, and we traveled home. I cried at every mile marker! Darrell had a great time and would call me on the phone and say, "Hi Aunt Donna, I am at Mom's house." He would be at Aunt Lynn's and knew how to push my button early. He was four that first time he stayed.

In Maryland, they had plenty of grandparents. My two grandmothers were still around for several years to enjoy both of the boys as was Pop Pop Clark. Pop Pop Clark insisted on calling Jared "Jericho", demonstrating a sense of humor I never saw as a child. And Nee Nee, who had married Townie, and he became a grandfather to them. Grandmom (Kitty) and Granddaddy (Alfred) were special for all of us. They lived close by and, as stated before, always available. Darrell and Jared learned country music riding in Granddaddy's truck when he was running errands. Once Darrell came home after a trip with Granddaddy singing, "All my Ex's Live in Texas." They loved the farm, and the many stories and treasures found there. Great Granddaddy (Avery) was there when they were boys and, of course, he told them how the pigs had eaten his two missing fingers long ago though he actually lost them in farming accidents. They took the boys shopping, out to eat, had sleepovers and went for rides and long walks. On vacation Grandmom sent postcards describing their adventures on pack trips or wherever their travels took them. When Grandmom and Granddaddy came home from vacation there was always a treasure for each grandchild and us adults, too. Grandmom and Granddaddy traveled often, visiting all fifty states. If Michael was traveling for work, they showed up so often just in time to save my sanity. They played ball with the boys, taught them life lessons and Grandmom even taught both boys to parallel park and took them for their driver's test. They came home from Fort Bragg the week Granddaddy died and had the honor of carrying their grandfather to his final resting place in their dress uniforms. The pride runs deep both ways.

Michael would sometimes travel for Aberdeen, and the boys and I stayed at home. When Dad was away we did fun things like stir our ice cream and camp out in our bedroom. The boys enjoyed the fact that Dad did secret stuff. The favorite line of Dad's was, "If I tell you I'll have to shoot you." One year he traveled to Las Vegas area every other month for a month at a time. Michael's parents were such a big help during that time. In February of 1988, I joined Michael for a long weekend in Las Vegas. From the snow on Mt. Charleston, to the hot sun of Death Valley, and the excitement of such a crazy city, we enjoyed every minute and put 800 miles on a rental car.

Life was so much easier when Dad was home. The boys always looked forward to Dad's return as the suitcase always held a special surprise for each of them and something for me, too. His many work trips to Florida brought them some interesting treats. When Michael wasn't travelling, the boys always looked forward to Dad coming home each evening from work. He typically arrived home at 5:10 PM, which is the time Darrell and Jared remember, and they were ready. Sometimes they jumped out to surprise him, as if he did not know they were in the house. It seems they always had something to show him.

Michael is the most patient of the two of us, so instructions often came from him. I must say, though, patience is not a strong virtue for either of us. After spending time running the two of them across the yard on bicycles, they began to catch on. Jared, though, only did things in his own timing, never ours, and accomplishes whatever he sets his mind to do. Darrell wanted to do everything yesterday. Both of them demonstrated their bike riding abilities for Dad after he arrived home from work. Darrell started at the top of the yard and attempted to ride over the bridge at the stream. He instead landed in the stream! On a different occasion, Jared started at the top of the yard and rode down toward the shed. He suddenly forgot how to use the brakes and nosed the bike directly into the shed. Fortunately, on both occasions, the injuries were minor. Welcome home, Dad.

These early childhood years are the years when my relationship with Candy and Dustin grew. I would babysit Dustin, and the three boys had many good experiences growing up. Candy and I often spent much time talking when she returned from work to pick up Dustin. The boys spent hours outside at the stream or in the woods and playing. When they were inside, you could find them in the attic or playroom with rarely a fight. Once an attic window was broken and I am still not sure which one actually broke the window. They all blamed each other. Since Jared was the youngest, he often got the blame, or they would blame Dustin after he went home. The boys did have many wars in that attic with GI Joe. Outside they built forts and usually ended up getting wet in the stream chasing frogs or building dams. Darrell and Dustin were caught more than once having a peeing contest. I do believe Dustin threw up in every car I had. Again, these are some years that I would not trade for anything. Candy has been a lifelong friend... together through it all.

Today I love pulling out toys from the attic or shed for the grandchildren. It is a treasure to watch them play with toys that were once their Dads'. Playmobile, Legos, GI Joe, blocks, balls, wagons, Big Wheel, trucks, scooters and sleds all bring back memories. The scooter reminds me of the Christmas Jared wanted it. He had asked for a red scooter, but all we could find was a purple one. So we convinced him he wanted a purple scooter, and then we found a red one while out shopping. We returned the purple one, bought the red one and slowly put the word red back into his thinking for a scooter. Parents must be creative, as I prefer not to use the word manipulative. Often I have been digging in the flower beds only to find an Army man or two, and I pause to smile and remember.

During these early childhood years, we also spent time with good friends. We would spend lazy summer days by the pool and often grilling hamburgers. The boys would play in the woods and streams. Darrell got quite a large, nasty gash in his knee that required several layers of stitches while catching crawfish in the stream by the Taylors. Darrell, Jared, Dustin, Philip and Bradford, sometimes joined by Marlene, Chris and Kelly, spent many a day swimming, playing and sledding together, too. A very memorable sledding day, they were sledding down the hill toward the pond with Darrell, Philip and Dustin stacked on a sled. Dustin bailed and the other two were hurled into a tree. As they crashed into that tree as we Moms watched, we were certain they were all dead. They all loved the outdoors. Some days we would load them all into our vehicle and go antiquing or to the farmer's market. We especially liked the antique shops with treasure boxes for the kids, and they always found something to add to their collections. Antiquing has remained one of my favorite things to do, and Jared still visits some of our favorite spots.

As a result of the antiquing and collecting family heirlooms over the years, both boys gained an appreciation for old things. Our house has several pieces of furniture with a very long family history. Many of those pieces will, hopefully, be passed down to one or both of them with their wives' approval and enjoyed with fond memories for many years to come.

Somehow, the boys never got lost or severely injured though they were able to wonder the woods freely on McCauley Road and spent many hours exploring, building forts and dams, getting wet in the stream, often at improper times and enjoying living in the country. More than once, as they were ready for church or we were just going away, the boys would run out the door to check for turtles or fish or had a sudden need to move a rock, hit the slippery grass and end up in the stream. Starting the process over of getting ready to go is not easy and stretched my patience often. As they grew and expanded their boundaries too far away for the sound of my voice, which was unusual as I can yell quite loudly, they could hear the old dinner bell ringing in the valley and knew to come home. From the large rocks in the back woods that could be a ship, mountain, hideout or actually a fox den, to the pond with fishing, row boating, ice skating and bon fires, they would travel and knew every inch of the woods. The Christmas they both got hockey skates, we had a frozen pond on that day and many days to follow. Their friends from school loved to come to the house and play endless games in the woods such as kick the can, ice hockey or campout in the yard or by the pond. I remember the summer Mrs. Daly called to say the boys "had come of age" as she saw them in the row boat with girls! Mom's pleasure comes in watching her children happy and thriving. Needless to say, they survived childhood. These are some sweet memories.

"I thank my God upon every remembrance of you." Phil. 1:3 KJV

Darrell and Jared were close and definitely brothers, yet so very different. Jared was usually smart enough to figure out if the action got his brother in serious trouble he would either avoid the action or be much more careful. Darrell would jump headlong into whatever the occasion, while Jared would examine the issues first. Darrell lives life without fear. Both bring us joy.

Darrell had an imaginary friend like his Mom did long ago. His friend was Elephant. Now Elephant was everywhere and we all got into the act. Since he was an Elephant, he lived under the front porch not in the house. Elephant could be seen playing in the stream, riding down the road in a truck with a perfect stranger or shopping at the mall. We could be on vacation somewhere and Michael would ask Darrell, "Isn't that elephant over there?" From that question quite a story could be spun. Elephant entertained us all for several years! Evidently Elephant has been blessed with a long life as Michael can still see him appear in odd places.

Jared was and still is the animal lover. Our close proximity to the road was not an ideal situation for some animals. So the pet graveyard in the back corner of the yard grew. We had numerous cats, but only Marino lived to be 20 years old. Marino arrived with her Mom, who we named Sandy, one stormy night at our front door. We told the boys the next time they wanted a pet to get together and pray instead of praying individually. We had chickens that Jared actually kept in his room on a couple of cold nights when they were young. We had sheep...now they were fun, but sheep are hard to raise. By the time you realize a sheep is sick he will probably die very soon. Jared even had a green iguana. When the iguana was active he could be insane, but usually you could find him sleeping on the highest point he could reach in the house. On one occasion, he was so angry because Jared was taking him inside on a summer day that he actually turned red. The iguana would sit on Jared's head, too. We had to remember to point him out to guests as to not scare them to death if he moved suddenly. And of course we had the occasional goldfish, hamster, gerbil and rabbit. He loved them all. I am thankful they did not all move in at the same time.

Those early years went by so quickly. I remember the days of spilled milk, muddy shoes, bloody accidents, and noisy boys. On those days in the middle of the chaos, there were times I would wonder if it would ever end. The frustrations on certain days seemed endless, but in truth, they are gone ever so quickly. Since then there have been many times I wished time would have slowed, but believe me in the middle of it all, I couldn't wait for them to move on to some other phase. Growing up comes too soon! But long before the growing up, came school days and teenagers. The properly written phrases of Hallmark cards do not always capture the reality of everyday living. Being a Mom is not for the faint of heart and perfection eluded me often. I am grateful for two sons that love me just like I am...flaws and strengths.

We told the boys often through the years that their brother was the best friend they could ever have. Brothers love through everything and forgive each other easily. Looking out for each other had been important during childhood, but would become more crucial through the teen and adult years. As they grew older, I always enjoyed watching them go do things together. Every time they left the house they got "the speech" from Mom. As children running around the house, I felt I had control over what was happening, but when they went out that door my control was gone. It is so easy to forget that is was never my protection they needed, but God's protection. One particular beach trip as teenagers comes to my mind. They went to Indian River Inlet in Delaware for the day. All I know about what happened is what they chose to tell me, but I saw the result when we finally got Jared to the hospital. The surf was very rough that day and Jared broke his leg. Evidently his big brother did not believe him when he said something was wrong until he saw the odd angle of his leg. Emergency room, calling Mom, plenty of drugs, driving home and on to the hospital for a few days stay are enough to make Mom queasy just remembering. I pray my sons are always friends!

Their lives continued to blend with mine as life goes on. As children they intertwined with my school teaching days. Darrell and Jared remained my most valued students. Our lives also stayed connected at home. We enjoyed going out to eat as a family. That was usually an event that occurred once a week. Their Dad always liked to take us for rides typically with a destination in mind. Jared usually enjoyed the rides, but Darrell only saw them as a means to an end and just wanted to reach the destination. As a result, Darrell often read to pass the time as we explored so when he was able to drive he sometimes had a difficult time with knowing the way. Jared made a good navigator for his brother as he always knew the way because he paid attention! If they were attentive, they could learn many roads because Michael rarely goes the same way twice and taught them that all roads lead home.

Running all these memories through my mind makes my heart sing. I may have regrets of things done or not done over time, but never regrets of time spent with my family.

> "Dost thou love life?
> Then do not squander time
> For that's the stuff life is made of."
> Ben Franklin

Dear Children,

If you have any regrets, learn from them. Then close that chapter of your life and never reopen it again. We cannot go back. Take what you learned and be thankful for the teaching moments in your life. Your Mom does well to remember this, too. Move forward without regrets for they are only weights that will hold you down and you were meant to soar.

Love, Mom

Chapter 6

Journey into Teaching

My education had pointed me in the direction of teaching and my dream and plan was to teach Physical Education and coach in a high school somewhere, but I allowed that dream to fall by the wayside. No regrets for that, as my life became so much richer than being that big coach could have ever brought. At this point in my life, I found myself with two little boys. Michael and I had decided that staying home with them was the most important work I could do. As I said earlier, the years of early childhood flew by.

When it was time for Darrell to begin school, we had a big decision to make. The choices were public school, homeschool (he and I would not survive), or Christian school. This was a major decision. We wanted our children to have the right influences with a well rounded education and made a choice. Because Darrell's birthday was in December, we were not too anxious to send him to school at age four. When the time came for kindergarten, Christian school was it. Darrell attended Harford Christian School in Dublin, Maryland from kindergarten through second grade. His kindergarten teacher, Maggie Meyer, was the perfect first teacher and we made good memories with Maggie in and out of school. We cannot forget the "fluffer nutter" sandwiches and the sledding in Churchville. She loved her students and Darrell looked forward to school. How thankful I was that his experience at school did not mirror my experience. It was very hard putting him on the bus that first day and I went home and cried. At least I had Jared to keep my day busy. Spending time with just Jared was something we both needed, and yet we both looked forward to Darrell coming home from school each afternoon. The best school story from those early school years is the time I got a phone call saying Darrell, as a first grader, had brought a dead shrew to school. Evidently, he had found it in the woods the day before and put it in his jacket pocket. At school he thought it would be fun to chase the girls with the shrew at recess. The school frowned upon this behavior. Sometimes I had to pretend I was angry. Darrell and Jared also played soccer in Harford County. These years began our connection to the Brooks family that obviously would became very important later. Alisha says she remembers noticing Darrell in line at school during those early years. The boys both played Little League baseball in the town of Rising Sun. Once again it was important to keep the boys well rounded by offering them choices of extra activities as they were available. It also kept us as a family involved in the community and created more circles.

During this time we made a change in churches. Leaving the church in Port Deposit area after so many years was hard, but we needed the change. We had passed a church so many times on our way to Quarryville, Pennsylvania and decided to visit. There we met a great group of people. To try to name these people and forget someone would not be fair. Some of them are dear friends to this day. These were all influences on our lives. This period of my life would require another book or the sequel that my family teases me about. I must speak of the Martins as they had a great influence on all our lives. Dave Martin was our pastor and affectionately became known as "Preacher". The value of these influences in our lives cannot be measured. The Martins and our church family walked us through many ups and downs. We are thankful for those years and the positive examples in our lives.

Jared had a hard time adjusting to this new church and social Darrell seemed to fit in well, but this church soon became home for all of us. We again became too busy and yet our family grew and learned during those years. My people-pleasing, insecure ways often flourished during these years as so often I struggled with being myself. Looking back at this period from this viewpoint, there are some things we may have changed, but that choice turned out to be what we believed to be best for our sons. Our choices did revolve around the entire family.

Most journeys do not form a straight line. We seem to have gone from point A to point B and now on to point C. For all of us, there comes a time for re-evaluation of where we are and where we want to be. The growing process should be lade with goals. Some goals are reached and others may lay dormant, often never fulfilled. The ultimate goal is to finish this life well. These years are all another circle of people and relationships that I am grateful to have had in my life and in the lives of our children who helped us strive for our goals. No regrets.

"The steps of a good man are ordered by the Lord..." Psalm 37:23 KJV

God is the only one who knows the end from the beginning and I trust him! I must be reminded of this often. Days lay ahead that God had been and still was preparing me for now.

Our church also had a school, and we made the decision to put the boys in their school. Darrell began third grade and Jared began kindergarten at our Christian school. We carpooled with the Andersons and soon that 17 mile trip became very familiar. We had even made the leap to a minivan! That was lowering my car standards and most parents find themselves making such changes to accommodate growing families.

In December of 1989, we had an unusually early winter. A few good size snowstorms made that drive even more exciting. On December 8th I had gone up the road to pick up the four boys because of an early dismissal. As we reached the Maryland/Pennsylvania state line, a truck slid through a stop sign directly in my path. The next few minutes are such a blur. Jeremy was riding shotgun and he was fine. Darrell was directly behind him and he, too, was alright. Jared had a large bump on his head from hitting the side window and Loren's face had hit the back of the second seat and he was bleeding. It was snowing hard and I was afraid for the kids. Someone stopped and the boys were given a warm place to stay in their vehicle. A Maryland snowplow stopped and as I sat on his running board, the driver kindly patched through a call to Michael at Aberdeen and to the Andersons. An ambulance arrived and at that moment I realized I was injured as my adrenaline was depleted. We were all transported to Harford Memorial Hospital and our families met us there. Loren and I had the worst end of the deal. His mouth had problems for a long time. I soon discovered that my patella was broken as a result of hitting the dashboard and the next eight weeks would be spent in a full leg cast and then surgery. A few days later Jared came to me and said, "Mom, I am sure thankful that wasn't a dump truck." Yes, Jared, so was I.

By the end of that first year the principal, Mr. Prater, offered me a job teaching a combined class of fifth and sixth grade. Up until this point in my life I had chosen to stay home with the boys once they were in the picture. Now we would be going to school together each morning and my world was being stretched. For the first few years, Connie Traub and I shared the day as I taught in the mornings. Connie took the afternoons. I learned many things about teaching from Connie and her experience as a teacher. I considered her my mentor. Lesson plans, grading and juggling time at home was often complicated, but we made it work. When Connie left the school, fearfully I took the whole day and now life was busier. Those teaching years were a challenge. A class size of 15 to 20 students was perfect. I had found a new rhythm as the boys and I went to school together every day. I even had a couple of teams to coach in volleyball and basketball during that time. I enjoyed my classes and, as I have mentioned before, many life experiences had prepared me for teaching in a small school.

Teaching brings notable experiences daily. Now anyone who has ever taken a class trip with a group of students knows anything can happen. One morning as we were headed to Aberdeen Proving Ground, a student threw up on the bus, and noticing it was orange, I assumed orange juice was his breakfast drink. I always tried to maintain my sense of humor at times like this, as it was my least favorite part of the job, so I joked with him about losing his orange juice. This story is remembered so vividly because the student replied, "Oh no, Mrs. Owens, I had cheese curls".

I broke my nose for the second time during those teaching years. We were playing basketball and one of the girls elbowed me in the nose. I had two black eyes for several days. Michael wrote a note to the principal asking that he keep a better eye on me. So many students I could write about at this point. I am grateful for each one and probably remember the difficult ones the best. They all taught me more that I could have ever taught them. Often in class I would tell them that I could write a book about them! Ok, the next book. I am grateful for ALL the students that passed through my classroom.

My students always enjoyed anything that made me seem like a real person and not someone who slept in the closet at school, reappearing each morning. They seemed amazed if I was ever tired, sick or emotional. When Michael would send a bouquet of flowers to my room with a card signed from my Lover, this brought many oohs and aaahs! I was actually human. Days when he visited school were even better. Michael encouraged and supported me in my teaching career and set a great example for Darrell, Jared and my students.

Our sons watched their fathers' actions carefully. Darrell, in his last two years of high school, would bring each girl and all female teachers a rose for Valentine's Day which made their day. When he graduated Jared picked up the practice. I am not sure if that was handed down spoken or unspoken. Hopefully, they have seen that the little things matter in relationships while watching their father and will incorporate them into their relationship with their wives. The time is now to put those things in practice.

Yes, I did have my sons as students and most of the time enjoyed it. You will need to ask them about how they felt having Mom as their teacher or of the pros and cons of being staff kids. When they were in trouble I was usually among the first to know. They did have their share of trouble and often rightly deserved. I enjoyed having Darrell and Jared at school as I didn't miss out on so much of their life. From the guys' point of view, I probably knew too much. So many times they were a big help in preparing the classroom or even giving suggestions as they moved on to other classrooms leaving my class behind.

There were a few perks to being staff kids, but probably more stresses. We got to school early, usually first, and left late, often last and the novelty of that wore off quickly. When they were injured on the playground or sick, I was there. For instance, the day Darrell caught a football and turned only to run directly into a tree and messed up that pretty face, I was there. Or the day after school when Jared and Jeremy were playing with a baseball bat and a basketball and Jared hit the basketball with the bat only to learn the two did not mix and have it bounce back to hit him in the head and required stitches, I was there to take him to the doctor. Learning can be hard. Often I was there for the squabbles and worked hard to stay out of playground politics as children grow in such situations. There were also pressures on us all. Life in the fishbowl can be difficult as I had learned long ago as a preacher's kid. The expectations were high, and the eyes upon us all were many. Just as in my life as a wife, mom and Nana, my experiences have formed me, so their life experiences have formed them into the men they have become.

My sons have made me very proud over the years. In reality, they were not perfect and got into their share of trouble, yet they grew into honorable young men. They maintained high grades in school, typically making the honor roll each marking period. They excelled in sports and I sure enjoyed watching them play soccer, basketball, flag football and baseball. As Mom, I was always there to cheer them on...often to their embarrassment. They appreciated Dad's quieter involvement much better. Darrell especially enjoyed the limelight of dramas and skits and Jared got in on the act, too. Jared and Darrell both sang in the choir and their talents in music are still being used today. They took piano lessons for a little while and both taught themselves to play the guitar and do it quite well. Jared plays his guitar, sings and leads the worship team at his church today. Darrell went on several missions' trips with our church and with his Granny and Pop, and has played the guitar and sang at their church. I am thankful for all their activities and mostly for their big hearts towards others.

Another important area to us was the work ethic of our sons. Living on McCauley Road was just what our boys needed. The best way to help keep a teenage boy out of trouble is to keep him busy and, therefore, tired when night comes. They learned to identify the correct tools for Dad and do small car repairs and so many other tasks around the house such as cleaning, laundry and cooking. If work was needed on the Owens farm, the boys were ready and accomplished many jobs for their grandparents. They put in many hours at home and on surrounding farms with Mrs. Daly, Mark Way, Allreds, Steve Haines, and the Coles on the horse farm through the years learning many skills including carpentry, roofing, stone work, animal care and farming skills.

During the teenage years came new adventures with vehicles, including speeding and even accidents. Every Mom worries about getting a phone call that her child has been in an accident. On one occasion Darrell and Jared were feeding the horses in Pennsylvania at the horse farm in the evening. I was home alone when a call came in that they were okay, but the truck was stuck across a rather large ditch. This was the days before cell phones and they had to rely on some kind person to allow them to call home. Actually, Jared had hit his head on the windshield and spilled a large bucket of feed, but not any serious injuries. Darrell told him he messed up his truck's windshield. Why do boys do this to their Mom when Dad is not home? Mark Way went to their rescue, and they were finally able to drive the truck home. On another day, Jared got into a little trouble with Dad as he was driving on a back road that was off limits in snowy weather. He slipped off the road, hit a bank and had a flat tire. He put the spare tire on his car and continued on to school. In his mind all was well and the tire was good for 50 miles or so. He went with some friends after school and went back that night to get into his car and head home when he had another tire was flat. So he did what boys do…call Dad. Perhaps you can see what was wrong with this story. Maybe he should have come straight home after school because of the first flat??? Another time Darrell had an accident on his way home from work, and gave his jeep a curled lip. I am thankful those phone calls did not hold any worse news. Remember to always begin your phone calls when possible to Mom with "I'm OK, but…

As a family we did things together. Our family vacations often took us to Indiana to visit my parents and sisters. We enjoyed these trips, but we knew we needed to be sure to include other places to enjoy as a family also. In the late 1980's my sister, Lynn, and family moved to Germany as missionaries. In 1992, we took a trip to Germany and surrounding countries to visit for two weeks. What a whirlwind trip as we visited several countries, and Dennis, Lynn, Michael, David and Kathleen packed the two weeks with much activity. In June 1995, we flew to Denver, rented a van and traveled from Estes Park to the Grand Canyon. We stayed on the North rim of the Canyon and enjoyed watching the boys build a lean to in the back of our cabin and finding it covered with fresh snow in the morning, consenting to Darrell climbing over the edge of the canyon to retrieve a stranger's hat and chase him down to return it, and watching Jared get so far ahead on a hike we asked a stranger coming towards us if he had seen him. We also visited several states with friends and family stops for 18 days. This included Four Corners, Las Vegas, and Independence Pass with plenty of snow, hikes and horseback riding and walked over the border into Mexico. Jared learned quickly that he was not from America but from the United States of America. Also, we have repeated often that Jared can sure ride a horse! We took many road trips close to home, as well as south to Florida and north to Maine, along with many times to the beach. I am grateful for plenty of good family memories of time spent together.

I planned to continue teaching even as the guys graduated, but I also struggled with some health issues. In 1992 after our trip to Germany I needed low back surgery, probably as a result of the earlier car accident. During this time, Mom again came to the rescue to help our household run smoothly in my absence. Soon Crohn's disease took control of my life for several years, as I lost 50 lbs in one month, required several medications and treatments, along with a strict change in diet. Eating was difficult and the boys' favorite line was "Is this something Mom can eat or is it good?" Michael did not appreciate this comment.

Suddenly a change of unimaginable consequences as our dear friends, Cindy and Steve, said goodbye to their son, Jason, on February 16, 2000. This is one of those times when the storm is raging and the calm has gone. Life was changing and the winds of change can be brutal. Then the year 2001 brought another big change with both of my grandmothers going to heaven within a month of each other that year. I still miss them. Death is a part of life we do not enjoy. As Christians we know we can look forward to being together forever in heaven where sorrow, pain or death will not be welcomed. It is comforting to know that God has welcomed home those who are His that have gone before us.

Psalm 116:15 KJV "Precious in the sight of the Lord is the death of His saints.

Chapter 7

Journey into an Empty Nest

An empty nest was not something I always looked forward to in the coming days. Michael and I had thought about the days when the boys were out of the house. Some thoughts were positive and others were negative. Perhaps it was time to change our focus. I had no idea how that would happen. There are some perks to having the house to ourselves, but it sure can be quiet. My emotions tend to show loud and clear as my family will attest to and the coming years would show my raw emotions often. As life would play out, the growing up years of our sons' lives would prove to have been the easy years. In Proverbs, God says he stores our tears in a bottle. My bottle of tears must be large. Tears of pride, anger, fear and pure joy flow easily.

Darrell graduated from high school in 1999 and Jared was in his senior year in 2001-2002, so I knew changes were coming. Both sons graduated from high school with honors, receiving awards for their outstanding character. Now was the time for them to move on. After all, this is one goal of parenting...to see your children go out and do something in this world. Darrell attended Bible College after high school and that ended abruptly...end of story. We all learned from that experience. Jared was finishing school and still working on the farms, when the world we all knew changed. Jared really did not appreciate his brother being away in college anyway, so when Darrell came home and began working a good job all was well. I certainly did not mind having them both at home again. It had been rather quiet when only our stealthy son was around. That boy has the ability to appear out of nowhere and he enjoys his mysterious entries.

But life does not stand still. September 10th was a different Monday night for us as Jared visited an Army recruiter to talk about some possibilities for after graduation. Then Tuesday, September 11, 2001 happened. I had an appointment with Dr. Weidner that morning as the events were unfolding. He told me a plane had hit one of the towers, but no other information was available. Heading to school after the appointment, I turned on the radio and the shock began to hit. After arriving at school, I told the other staff what was happening. We turned on the TV and watched as so many perished on that day. This day was about to change not only the United States of America, but my family as well. Jared said that day secured his determination to enter the Army. He enlisted with plans to leave that summer after graduation. Not long after Jared's enlistment, Darrell also decided to join the Army. You see Darrell and his Dad had a sit down, man to man talk, as Darrell had a good job, was hard working, but had no real sense of direction and no place to advance. Way too often he reminded me of myself. I am so thankful for the wise counsel of their Dad, Grandparents and even Sgt. Perkins during this time. After Darrell enlisted, I told Sgt. Perkins he was finished here as I had no more sons. My emotions were overflowing…a mix of pride and fear as my sons answered the call.

Jared was on delayed entry as he was a senior in high school. Darrell would be entering boot camp first. But as usual, Darrell finds exciting twist to put on any story. He decides to fall in love! Alisha Marie Brooks had entered his life and is still the best thing to ever happen to him. Now remember, this is from my perspective as Mom looking on as my son falls in love. Plenty of girls had chased him and they always tried to win me over to become their ally in obtaining my son. I was not an easy take. This was not true of Alisha. She came into all of our lives and did not try to be anyone other than herself. This new found relationship was different from the start.

Darrell came home talking about this Brooks girl one night after spending time talking to her as she worked at Steak and… We all knew the family and Darrell told us he had searched far and wide for his girl only to find she was living a few miles away (at one point even on McCauley Road) all his life. From my angle, the romance was fast. They love to tell you the story about the first night at the Brooks house when Darrell did not come home and it was well after midnight. My thought as Mom was, Dennis Brooks is going to shoot this kid! Yes it is true, I showed up there in the middle of the night in my pajamas and robe. Mom always tries to make a memory!

Darrell would be leaving soon for basic training, so they did move rather quickly. Watching young love blossom is so fun. They were silly and busy and growing very close. I still laugh at the sight of them emerging from the basement inside the same coat. Alisha was the spark that until now Darrell had never known and his Dad and I could not be happier. Alisha often joked that she dated me more than my son during those early Army days. We were impressed with the maturity of a young lady that would commit to a man about to head off to the Army and most certainly war. She joined us on many road trips with our destination being a military base. Often her sister, Susie, would come also and once again my life was filled with not only youth, but now with girls. In January of 2002, we took the first of many trips and saw Darrell off from MEPS. I am not sure which was the most difficult sometimes…saying goodbye or watching Alisha say goodbye.

Darrell's graduation from Basic Training took us all to Fort Benning, Georgia. After Basic, Darrell left for Fort Sam Houston, San Antonio, Texas, for Medic training. Jared was to graduate from high school in May, and Darrell really wanted to come. Somehow, he wanted to surprise everyone from Alisha, Jared, his Dad and all the Grandparents. He was able to get a pass and flew to BWI. Marlene was the only other person in on the plan. She picked him up at the airport and dropped him off in the upper part of the yard while everyone was getting ready to leave for graduation. I met him at the back gate of our garden and took him inside. I thoroughly enjoyed watching the shock on faces. First Jared, then the grandparents were so surprised. None were as surprised as Alisha, coming down the stairs to find Darrell standing in the living room. I still enjoy that memory and am so sentimental about the garden gate. They went out the door on the porch for an alone moment, and Dad came down from getting ready still unaware of what was happening. When he looked on the porch his first comment was, "Son, are you AWOL?"

The weekend went by quickly and soon Darrell was on his way back to Fort Sam. Jared, Daniel and I left for Spanish Wells, Bahamas, for a week. This trip was wonderful and I do not take it for granted that my son and his friend were willing to spend their graduation trip with me. You realize that I paid the way for Jared, so how could he refuse. They were given their space, but I also had the privilege of spending much time with them. I tried to soak in every ounce of that time before Jared would leave for Basic Training. This was not my picture of an empty nest. Our nation at war had not crossed my mind.

The week before Basic, Jared and Alisha flew to Texas to spend a long weekend with Darrell and after returning, he, Alisha and Susie went to Ocean City, Maryland for a day. Remember, one of my pleasures as Mom is watching my children enjoy themselves. I did not have to be a part of every moment to be able to do that. Observing from a distance often makes me smile. On June 18th we took Jared to MEPS and said our goodbyes as he left for Fort Jackson, SC. This was only the beginning of hard goodbyes, as I cried for a long time that day knowing he was leaving, but also knowing there were harder days ahead.

July brought Darrell heading to jump school and back to Fort Benning. I was excited for him, but could not decide if I wanted to know before he jumped or after he jumped. His first jump was July 11th and somehow over the years I learned to enjoy his jumping out of perfectly good airplanes. Once again, I was a proud Mom as he earned his jump wings. He was so excited to be able to jump on the Army's time. He fell in love with jumping a year or so before. He and Ryan Foster went for a jump unknowing to us until he popped in the video upon his return. Now in the 82nd Airborne, he was jumping on a regular basis. He was assigned to Fort Bragg, North Carolina in the 82nd Airborne Division.

Michael and I actually went on a road trip alone that July to visit my family in Indiana and then on to Michigan for Ryan and Jen Foster's wedding. For some reason I did not like to be away from home while the guys were serving in the Army, as if my being home helped in any way. I was never comfortable when they were traveling until I knew they had reached their destination. A strange "mom" thing...

Darrell had talked to us of his desire to marry Alisha and we fully approved. He made an appointment with her Dad after his return from Fort Benning and asked for Alisha's hand in marriage. I was nervous for him that day, because that is another thing mom's do. I knew my son was not only marrying Alisha, but gaining another family, too. Dennis and Dianna love Darrell, and Susie has become the little sister he never had. He was also gaining two more "brothers" in Tim and Jason. What a comfort to know that another family loved my son and considered him a part of their family. And I was glad to finally be getting another woman in the family and a special daughter-in-law as she and I had bonded already. Darrell popped the question and gave her a diamond on August 7, 2002. We knew when they left the house that day what his plan was as he took her to the Lighthouse in Havre de Grace, but I was anxious for their return to know for sure Alisha said yes. We gave them an engagement party at the Dudecks. At this party was one of the few squabbles Alisha and I ever had, and I do not even remember what it was about. My struggles were with wanting everything to be perfect as the mother-in-law thing was brand new and I had so many unspoken fears about the future. Darrell headed back to Fort Bragg and all was well with Alisha and me.

Alisha had a short period of time to plan a wedding and she and her Mom always included me in the planning. Alisha has been a treasure from the start. We all continued our trips to military bases as the training for each son continued. The trips often included hotel stays and many meals out. Michael and I, along with Alisha and Susie, headed to Fort Jackson for Jared's graduation. Susie was a great addition and always noted any wrong turn Michael made on the trips. I am not sure Susie ate anything other than chicken fingers on any of the trips. This drive meant we needed to drive past Fort Bragg. What a painful section of road for Alisha! Darrell was early in his Army career and the times we could see him at that point were limited. In South Carolina, we saw Bob and Mary Ellen and all of us attended Jared's graduation.

Tears flowed as my youngest marched past us, as another proud moment was experienced as mom. From there, Jared left for aviation training in Fort Eustis, VA. We then drove back to Fort Bragg for our first visit to see Darrell. Once again it was pure joy for me to watch Darrell and Alisha together, but my heart had moments of fear for them and what lay ahead. During this period of time, watching them say goodbye was the hardest part. How many tears can a mother cry?

Somehow, in all of this, Michael was still working at Aberdeen and I was teaching. This particular year it was kindergarten. I decided to fill a last minute need the school had for the new school year. This would be the first and the last time for me to teach this class, but I really did enjoy it. I had so many other things to focus on. The schedule was a little less demanding and I managed to juggle it all.

In October, Jared came home on a three day pass from Fort Eustis on the bus. Now this was quite an experience for me in just picking him up. Michael had used the bus in his Army days, but I had never been to a bus station. Baltimore station is not exactly the glamour spot of the city. We learned his bus was delayed after we arrived and Michael and I spent most of the night playing cards and people watching. Even a country girl can pick out a pimp in the crowd. I must say the wait was interesting. Jared arrived safely, and we enjoyed his company for a few days.

In November, we had a bridal shower for Alisha and it was well attended from all sides. Her Mom and sister had planned it at Harford Christian School. Whenever Dianna is involved with a party it is a guarantee the food will be outstanding and abundant. It was such fun watching Alisha open all those gifts and my thoughts jumped ahead to their future. I had the feeling that day that she felt as I did so many years earlier about the kitchen. We all learn in time and today she is a great cook, because she really was listening and watching her mother all those years!

Thanksgiving brought both boys home for the weekend and I would always wonder where they would be next year at this time. Sometimes it is hard to just live the moment knowing we have no control over anything else. I worked hard to stay focused on this time at home and not think too much. The excitement of youth kept me going. One day Darrell and Alisha dressed in his Army uniforms and took a trip to Rising Sun. They were carefree, and I worried that she was impersonating an Army soldier. The difference a little age makes!

One of my favorite family times to this day is playing games. Skip Bo, Golf, Phase 10, 9 Up 9 Down, Hand and Foot, and What's Wild are among the favorites. We all like to remind Jared that he holds the record in Phase 10 for the highest score when the point is to have the lowest scoreJ. Many times you will find a score card on the refrigerator of our last round of games with the winners' name circled. It disappears quickly unless I am the winner. We are a competitive group. Playing games, we all laugh, yell and often demonstrate our various personalities while just plain having fun! We all tend to jump on the one who is down and we never forget…a hard crowd that loves each other dearly. Cheating may be possible in our group so if you play with us, stay sharp. And never play with Alisha and Susie sitting side by side or allow Alisha to use a glass top table. I will play games any and every night if one will join me and now I have a grandson who loves to play games and enjoys beating me in Sorry or one of the many other games he plays, and our second daughter-in-law, Julie, also brings her competitive nature to the table. There I go getting ahead of myself again.

Darrell headed back to Fort Bragg and Jared back to Fort Eustis. Darrell's agenda was full as he prepared for his soon to be wife. He found an apartment in Spring Lake that was quite nice. The important part was to please Alisha and for her to feel safe, as is always true when you take a wife! Some great memories were made in that apartment for all of us, from game playing to goodbyes.

Darrell and Alisha were married in December 21, 2002, and how proud we were of the choice our son had made and the daughter-in-law we were getting. All the guys gathered to our house on December 19th. Jared, Dustin, Jason Prokop and Darrell enjoyed each other's company. The Army guys even went for a morning run on wedding day. My family arrived and we had a large gathering for the rehearsal dinner with Alisha's family joining our family and the wedding party. The wedding was beautiful as Darrell and Alisha enjoyed each other throughout the ceremony. One of Darrell's youngest cousins, Benjamin, was in the wedding. I watched from the front seat as he grew very pale and grabbed him before he passed out. Pastor Martin and Dad performed the ceremony. We all had a good time at the reception at Willow Valley, though it was short, as they needed to get to the airport. They left for the Bahamas honeymoon and so began their new life. Once again, I was never more proud or teary than when watching them leave the reception. Alisha again demonstrated her commitment to our son and this marriage, knowing she would be leaving her family in Maryland and moving to North Carolina. Their time in the apartment would be short as Darrell would be sent to Iraq soon.

I must insert a note about Jason Prokop. Jason was a California boy. He was a good friend to Darrell and Alisha and also helped Jared. We all had enjoyed his company over the Army years. He, like Darrell, was an Army medic and Darrell's battle buddy. One time when we were in North Carolina, Alisha and I allowed Jason to practice his blood draws on us and he would actually take blood. A very good memory was made! Jason got out of the Army and married and became a San Diego Police Officer. He has two sons similar in ages as our oldest grandsons. On October 1, 2011, Jason was on his way home from work one night and stopped on a bridge to help a lady. He was hit by a car and killed that night. Helping others was the way he lived and then died. It is our honor to have known Jason.

Christmas was different for us all this year. The Brooks' family was without Alisha and our family without Darrell, leaving Jared sitting alone on the steps for the traditional Christmas morning picture. We had the hope that one day we would have them both home for Christmas. This year they spent Christmas in the Bahamas and found themselves homesick on Christmas day. After coming home for a few days, the newlyweds headed to NC on the 29th to enjoy the weeks together before the next phase of Army life. Again, my mind wonders to what next year will hold as I try to remind myself to enjoy the moment.

January, 2003, Michael and I load up the car with mostly Darrell and Alisha's stuff as would be the case from now on. We have hauled large pieces of furniture down that road for them. From there, we took

Jared back to Fort Eustis to finish his aviation training. We drove back to Fort Eustis the end of January for Jared's graduation from school and on January 22, his Dad pinned his aviation wings on his chest. Jared had just graduated at the top of his class. This mother's heart was very enlarged by this time! Jared headed from there to Fort Benning for jump school, and again did I really want to know every scheduled jump?

Proverbs 3:5a KJV "Trust in the Lord with all your heart..."

Both families headed to North Carolina to say our goodbyes to Darrell. This was only one of many trips to Fort Bragg as this part of the journey began. Actually, Michael has counted 35 trips to Fort Bragg alone!

SONS TO WAR

February 12, 2003, is a day my mind will never forget, but at the same time the details are gone. Darrell departed that day for parts unknown to all of us, yet we knew the ultimate goal would be Iraq. Now the praying, waiting, watching the news, ignoring the news, and praying some more was the daily routine. Alisha, once again, came home to her family and us. Alisha should be and would be the first one he contacted when possible and she and I had an understanding. We would always let the other know when news came from Darrell. Alisha was faithful to let us know when she heard from Darrell, and having the one he loved so much around us helped to keep me going. So often I am asked how I did this and my answer is always the same. God brought me through and the details I really don't always remember.

This day of technology is such a blessing compared to the families waiting on news during any previous wars. If Darrell contacted us, we would let Alisha know because we had a deal. First of all, we thought it was most important that Darrell and Alisha communicate as much as possible. If he only had one chance to call or short period of time on the computer, he should spend it with Alisha. If Alisha or I got a letter from Darrell we would share it with each other. Well, I shared all of my letters and she chose carefully the parts to read to me. We spent many hours reading letters out loud to each other, and then privately reading and rereading his letters. God always seemed to know when this mothers' heart could not stand it for another moment, and Darrell would get in touch with us. His Dad and I felt as though we followed him through the sands of Iraq and into Baghdad daily. Michael, being the detail person, would have a map of Iraq handy. We prayed for him and knew we could only trust God and his plan for our son. Alisha may not understand the joy and comfort she brought to us by just being around. She was, and still is, a special gift to us all.

Jared completed jump school in February, earning his jump wings and came home until the middle of March for a break. We actually had several large snowstorms that year and Jared was a big help getting the heavy snow off the roof of our house. The guys have no problem helping around the house when they are home.

By that time, we had word that Darrell's unit had gone into Iraq and they were headed toward Baghdad. Letters trickled home and I would laugh, cry, and imagine the scenes he tried to paint with a pen, rereading the letters often. Still, to occasionally hear his voice was the best, for in that voice I knew he was well. Darrell also kept a journal of his days into Iraq and shared them with us. When we received a section of journal we knew he was telling us his gut feelings. He told of "still driving —no time for sleep." "The thing that is most noticeable about Iraq is it is ugly. At night we could see distant oil well fires and when daylight finally broke all we could see was sand and dirt." He told of close calls and also of calmer times. He was amazed to be walking in lands he had read or heard about in Bible times. He bemoaned the fact that his unit was not able to jump into the Baghdad airport as Turkey had not allowed the use of their airspace. He recalled a church service they held in the desert. He told of sleeping under the stars and seeing Orion and being homesick. Yes, this all tugged at this Mom's heart. Darrell told us later of a time that really hit him hard. A soldier was brought in and didn't make it. Darrell told of being the one to remove the wedding ring of a soldier to place with his personal effects and realizing that his family did not yet know. Of course, his thoughts went to Alisha. These were painful days.

On one occasion something happened that reminded me of their youth and confidence that all would be well. Darrell was riding around Baghdad after the city had been taken by our troops in an open humvee. Those early days were very different from the later days. He had asked Alisha to send a video camera so he could capture the city for our viewing. First of all, could you really send a video camera to Iraq and expect it to make it? Secondly, did I really want to see it first hand from my son? From my perspective the answer to both of these questions was no. Mom was wrong on the first account. The camera did make it. On the second account, my answer was still no and everyone thought it best if Mom did not see some of these pictures until Darrell was safely home. Good choice, children!

We had settled into a routine, if there is such a thing when war is happening and your son is in the middle of it all. Jared was being stationed at Fort Bragg and Darrell's friend and battle buddy, Jason Prokop, was there to show him around.

April brought some new twists. Alisha needed to take care of some business in North Carolina, and Michael and I volunteered to take her down, which meant we could visit with Jared, too. Now it is Mom's turn to add another twist. I was having some neck issues and thought they were improving, but the day before we were to head south I could not lift my left arm. Dr. Weidner sent me to Dr. Boulos that day who told me I needed emergency surgery on Saturday or else lose use of my arm permanently. Michael and Alisha made a blitz trip to North Carolina, Jared was granted leave to return for my surgery, and Alisha contacted Darrell through the Red Cross. Alisha was hoping they would agree it was serious enough to have Darrell come home, but that didn't work. Darrell's emails show that was an anxious time for him wondering what was happening at home. Surgery went well as they fused C - 4,5,6. They found a substitute for school and my recovery began, as Mom came in to help so Michael could return to work. Michael made another trip to Fort Bragg to get Jared back to duty and life continued.

In July, Alisha and I made another trip to North Carolina for her to take care of business and the apartment and, of course, we visited Jared. As usual, she and I always had time for some shopping. Jared's aviation unit was in full preparations for going to Iraq by September. In August, we talked to Darrell a little more as he had a break in Qatar. Again, I was not sure I wanted to know too many details of his days in Iraq as Jared was headed there very soon. Then the weekend of August 28th, Michael and I headed to Fort Bragg to watch Jared leave for Iraq. Ok, God, what are you doing? He promised not to give me any more than I could handle! One war, two sons, countless prayers!

Somehow as Mom, I just went through the day to day, struggling to remain in the calm eye of the storm. Darrell and Jared were not separated by very many miles in Iraq, but circumstances never allowed them to see each other and to only talk maybe once. My mind could not help but go to a dark place sometimes, and picture Alisha coming with bad news or that dreaded Army vehicle coming in our driveway with uniformed men walking to my door. I had told both of our sons that they were heroes for serving their country and to please take care and keep their heads down. But they had a job to do and, knowing them, I knew they would do it well no matter the cost. They are the kind of men I would want to have my back. Thankfully, most days I was able to stay focused and trust that God knew exactly what He was doing. I had Michael and I had Alisha! I found outlets for my concern by advocating for our troops in our county. Numerous newspaper articles were written with some that included excerpts of Darrell's experiences in Iraq. We formed a group of mostly Moms that had a yellow ribbon tree placed on the square in Rising Sun and gathered names of local troops serving our nation. We had a couple of prayer vigils in town for all the troops, and when anyone came home we tried to be sure they received their ribbon from the tree as a reminder that their community had remembered. Care packages were another way to stay active in our troop's lives and many local businesses participated. It was all energy well spent. The guys loved the care packages not only from me, but from so many others, some of which they did not even know. Now I am getting letters from not only Darrell, but also Jared. Jared speaks of gray skies and being busy with the Blackhawks. He also wants to be able to call home, but the phones are not the best at this point. He says the sand is so hard on the helicopters, especially the blades. By November, Jared was sleeping on a mattress and thought it was wonderful. He still had hopes of seeing his brother. I had just sent a box to them both with a Christmas tree and Jared reports having his up and the gifts under the tree with a promise not to open anything until Christmas morning. I recall receiving a picture of his little tree with the gifts by his cot with bullet pocked concrete surrounding him.

The holidays of 2003 were extremely different for us all. I had sent our sons those little trees and plenty of packages to open for Christmas along with some of their favorite cookies and even the traditional Christmas Eve gift, but missed them terribly. Alisha again brought joy to our Christmas day by spending some time with us. Michael's Dad had been sick this year and was in Calvert Manor to recover. So in every way Thanksgiving and Christmas was just not the same. How grateful I was to hear their voices on each holiday, and how difficult it was to fight back the tears. I did not want to waste my talk time with them blubbering, so I held back most of the tears until we hung up the phone. Those conversations lingered in my thoughts until it was finally time for the next call. We would try to get so much news into each phone call and hang up every time realizing something I forgot to say. Three words were the most important..."I love you". Often I would say those words first just in case our conversation was cut off in the middle as sometimes the phone lines would go dead. They both always wanted to convince us they were well. I knew that my sons had left as boys and would be coming home as men. One phone call from Jared kept me awake for the rest of the night. Because of the time difference we often received their calls around 2 or 3 am. This night Jared was fighting to keep control. A Chinook had gone down full of soldiers heading home. His task was recovery. No one survived that crash. He said one of the most difficult tasks was picking up the strewed pieces of those soldier's lives from the soldiers' bags, knowing they would never be returning home. The hard stories of war are theirs to tell if they choose, not mine, but war changed them forever, and it touched this mother's heart in a way nothing else ever did. My days of protecting my sons from the horrors this world can hold were over, and I often heard the change in their voices.

In January, 2004, we got word that Darrell's unit was coming home. On January 26th, they moved out of Iraq into Kuwait. One son out of harm's way and was soon to come home to his anxious wife and family. Meanwhile, Jared remained in Iraq in Fallujah. On January 30th, he turned 20 years old. This is not where most of the young men that age are in their lives. His maturity was not easily gained. Part of me remained in Iraq for now, as part was coming home.

These next events are indescribable, as we all anxiously awaited Darrell's arrival. The Owens/Brooks clan headed to Fort Bragg. Watching the sheer joy and excitement on Alisha's face was overwhelming. February 6, 2004, Darrell and his unit marched off that airplane onto the Green Ramp to a building vibrating with the band playing and people cheering. My emotions come to the surface as I write and remember that day. Finally home! Finally holding Alisha in his arms and finally as Mom to get my long awaited hugs. All I had longed for was to touch him and know he was home. I shed so many tears of sheer joy that day just watching the scene around me in the building that included Darrell and Alisha and so many other soldiers. I can't imagine that I will ever forget that day. Alisha and I had shared a time in history that solidified our relationship and changed us all. We all went to dinner at the place of Darrell's choice...Olive Garden and focused on the moment! That evening we parents all said our goodbyes and headed back to Maryland. Darrell and Alisha would come soon as he would have a 30 day leave and many people who wanted to see him. They spent time in Maryland with a big welcome home party at the Brooks' house, flew to Indiana to visit family and then, on March 1, back to Fort Bragg for some well deserved alone time for the two of them. Darrell was home and my world was halfway back together.

Jared's time in Iraq was coming to an end soon. On March 13th he called from Kuwait. Now I could breathe deeply again. Both of my sons had made it safely out of Iraq. I do not know why, but God had been merciful. It is painful to think of the Moms whose sons did not come home. Those units standing in front of cheering families were not complete because of war. For them, I also do not know why, and I weep with you. These are questions not to be answered on this side of heaven. All I know is that God loves us so much that he allowed his own Son to die for us, even though we do not deserve it. This means God understands even when I do not. The only way to survive is to trust. The prevailing winds can be fierce.

April 7, 2004, we once again were standing at the Green Ramp this time in the middle of the night as the troops marched in to hungry arms waiting hugs. For all the things I did not understand there was one thing I knew. I knew one result it should bring from me. I had to stop and say "Thank you, Lord". I did not deserve this pleasure, but I was thankful. We were together again for now, and I was still working on enjoying the moment. This was a time of celebration!

For the moment life was back to normal. At least normal as far as the Army went. Jared had his 30 day leave and enjoyed a well-deserved break. Darrell and Alisha were adjusting to married life, settling into Fort Bragg area, and we all traveled up and down the road from North Carolina to Maryland easily. In July, Darrell earned his Sergeant Stripes. Tim (Alisha's brother) and Laura were married that month and we all enjoyed the celebration. Family weddings have a way of bringing us all together in a joyful time.

Michael's Dad was back in Calvert Manor. My father-in-law was the backbone of the Owens family, and his illness was difficult to handle. He had always been the fixer and now he needed fixed. I officially resigned from teaching citing a variety of reasons with no intentions of going back. Life moved on.

So if your picture of an empty nest is quiet as my picture once was, remember, it could be the opposite. Even when they are grown, our children still need us, but now we only step in with advice when we are asked. Our children are always our children, yet spending time with them changes. They can run, but they can't hide...Mom will find them and promises to visit and hopefully always has enough sense to know when to keep her mouth closed and when it is time to go home.

Christmas once again would be complete for me, having both sons and Darrell's wife sitting on the steps on Christmas morning. Life continued on…yet none of us knew this would be the last Christmas with Michael's Dad. Alfred was very sick after the New Year, and he passed away on February 2, 2005. This was a man who influenced us all and I was privileged to call him my father-in-law. One of his favorite lines was "keep the forked end down" and we all were trying. His was a life well-lived and sorely missed.

After his funeral service that day, as we were leaving the farm, my phone rang. Darrell and Alisha had gone back to the cemetery looking for the shells from the twenty-one gun salute as Alfred had been laid to rest with full military honors having served in the occupation forces in Japan at the close of World War II. The snow had been pretty deep and Darrell pulled off the road and found himself stuck. Having just lain to rest a man he loved and respected, his emotions were raw. Not being one to express those emotions very well, he had held them in for the past few days. Now they were about to flood Calvert. He was furious after getting stuck and called his Dad to bring a chain. We did not see or hear the beginning of this screaming session, but when we arrived, Alisha was sitting on a tombstone alone and Darrell was storming around still angry. Alisha told Michael to please take her home and she meant to her parents house. Michael kindly told her no and as she climbed into the car with him. Once Darrell's car was out of the deep rut he said he would drive to our house. When we reached home, I think I treated them like two little children by telling them to go up to Darrell's old room. Now I do not recommend that a parent become a marriage counselor for their children except for an emergency. This was an emergency. Alisha has told me that day could have easily gone the other way and saw it as a turning point for them and told me that I had to share these events. I forced them to talk it out and encouraged Darrell to finally shed those tears. Real men need to learn how and when to cry. Being left alone they had to deal with the situation by talking it out. They were trapped…no running and no quitting. Always talk it out no matter how difficult. Running away will not solve any issues. Couples need to learn how to fight and then enjoy the making up.

Darrell, Alisha and Jared once again stayed around for a few days to help with some farm work and then all returned to Fort Bragg once again. On the farm we brought out some of the Owens' guns to have a little target practice. I soon learned that my daughter-in-law is not one to contend with!

In March 2005, Alisha and Darrell bought a house in Sanford. Alisha's parents went down to help them paint and get ready to move. We joined in on the fun and saw another big step in our son's life. Home ownership...or does it own you? It certainly makes more sense than paying rent and Alisha and Darrell made it home.

Michael was getting close to retirement from Aberdeen Proving Ground. This year he and I attended several classes together to help us prepare financially for what was ahead. Michael's traveling days were over for Aberdeen and we were starting to enjoy more time together. We spent time with his Mom helping out with the farm. She had always wanted to chop the bottoms off all those holly trees and this was the year to accomplish that task. His Mom continued to be a hard worker and still mowed the grass and made sure Michael kept the low limbs trimmed. If a limb was low enough to knock off her hat it meant it was in need of a trim.

In June, we took Michael's Mom to North Carolina for the grand tour of Fort Bragg and to see exactly what her grandsons were doing. Grandmom actually sat in one of Jared's Blackhawk as she visited her grandsons' units. She noticed a shortage of chairs at Darrell and Alisha's house for the kitchen table and bought them some folding chairs to use as extras. She took us all out to dinner at Texas Roadhouse for Michael's birthday, and we ended up getting the meal free because of the poor service. She had a drink spilled on her at Andy's Restaurant when Alisha slipped and hit the table. We were all there for Alisha's baptism that weekend, too. Activity and excitement seemed to follow Grandmom for those few days and we all enjoyed her very much. I must say she travels well!

In July, Jared had a three month deployment to the Bahamas chasing drug runners in the Blackhawk. We heard a few of these tales, but the good times were fishing and grilling the catch. Having Jared in the Bahamas was very different for me than having him in Iraq for obvious reasons even though the threat was real when on duty.

In August of this year, I made a decision...not a good decision. The board asked me if I would come back to school for a couple of years to help keep the consistency in school after many changes had occurred. Just a reminder to you...it is ok to say no. I wish I had learned that little word much earlier in life. Try it sometime, as it is refreshing or so I have heard.

My Dad was beginning some major medical issues and spent much time in the hospital this particular year. At this time, he and Mom were living in northern Indiana near my little sister and family. Dad was diagnosed with NPH and had a shunt inserted in his head at a Chicago hospital. Dad also began having mini-strokes. Mom, on the other hand, was still in good health and full of energy. Long distance between my parents and me is difficult. The aging of parents is never easy.

School was balanced with sons reaching milestones and parents getting older. Darrell re-enlisted in the Army on September 15, 2005. In October, Jared went to NCO school and I needed to take a trip to Indiana to visit my parents. Now, why did I say yes to go back to school?

Michael was, and still is, a very romantic guy. Even while the boys were still at home he would come up with creative dates. One time he had his parents babysit and then sent me on a very detailed scavenger hunt. After some shopping and gathering, I was led to a nice hotel where we had dinner and spent the night. Almost every June, he takes me on a small trip, usually keeping the destination secret, as we celebrate our anniversary. This particular year we dated through the alphabet. Michael got the idea from Darrell and Alisha, even though I do not think they have tried it yet. Our first date was at the Avenue in Whitemarsh. Some dates were a restaurant or hike and others were an overnight. The Z date was to Zwaandel Inn in Lewes, DE and a visit to Zale's for some new jewelry. We run away often and most of the time it is his plan and kept a secret until we arrive at the destination. An unplanned lunch or dinner date is always welcomed by me. Unplanned was not often possible when the boys were small, but now it works very well! This man keeps the excitement and wonder in our marriage of 40 years and running. Others would benefit from his example. Once again, I hope my sons are paying attention.

A good marriage is a balancing act, as the years bring new challenges. When we were young and going in so many directions, we took time for us. As time went on and children took more time, we still took time for us. Then we began chasing children around the country and helping out with our parents as they grew older and we still took time for us. I pray that in our later years as time is even more precious, we still take time for us.

Sons, always take time for the most precious gifts ever given you... your family.

Christmas once again found everyone home for the holidays. I love this time of the year, but must warn myself that my perfect picture of how to spend this time will not always happen. Enjoy the moment, enjoy the moment...stop worrying about next year before this one is even over.

Fun stuff is so important. I love fun! In February, we went to Fayetteville and took Darrell and Alisha to the circus. This was Alisha's first circus and I get such pleasure watching her have fun. We did it all...hats, noses that light up and cotton candy. We enjoyed time with them even before grandchildren!

Both of the guys were busy with the Army and Jared was preparing for his unit to deploy to Afghanistan soon. He spent a few weeks at Fort Carson for mountain training in the Blackhawk. Darrell had proven himself as a leader and Jared, too, was becoming a leader. I enjoyed hearing Darrell tell of watching his brother give instruction to others as they prepared for flight on the Blackhawk. Darrell was proud of his little brother and what he had become. Jared had fallen in love with the Blackhawk. On one occasion Jared and Darrell actually jumped together out of the Blackhawk. In April, Jared went to Fort Polk for more training in preparation for deployment.

Breaks from the routine are so important and we have tried to demonstrate that for our family. Physical activity on the farm can rejuvenate for other task. One such task was to be the last time that Michael and the boys would trim a tree known as the bonsai tree on the

Owens' farm. The tree is very unusual as it has gnarly branches and had grown quite large. It was a day to remember and none of them really wants to do it again. Darrell and Alisha went on a missions' trip with their church to Canada on one break, also. Breaks come in many forms and are necessary for survival.

A major life changing event was about to happen, and the announcement was a day to remember. Darrell and Alisha came to the house with a package for me to open as they were here for her brother, Jason and Liz's wedding. Now it wasn't Christmas, my birthday or even Mother's Day. Alisha had her camera ready. I opened a Willow Tree grandmother and child and began to cry. Our first grandchild was on the way! I actually ran out on the front porch and yelled my news to the world. Michael was thankful we live in the country. This was life changing. I could not wait until this little one's arrival and today you must forgive me for my ability to talk about my grandchildren. They are the most beautiful and smartest grandchildren ever born.

Darrell was off to Yuma for more jump training. I was back to school. I guess that letter was destroyed and everyone, including me, pretended I really wanted to be teaching school fulltime, and I did enjoy the classroom again. A paycheck meant I could buy baby stuff, and that I did. Jared continued to train and we were still traveling up and down the road. Jared got in on the act of the upcoming baby by purchasing the unborn nephew his first shoes, and we brought the car seat and stroller. This was also the year we actually got Cable TV and our sons welcomed us to this century.

Thanksgiving brought everyone home again. Cindy helped me give Alisha a baby shower and we had quite a crowd. We had the shower up the hill from our house at the Mt. Pleasant UMC and had so much fun. Christmas brought that hint of sadness as we all knew Jared was leaving in January for Afghanistan, but a baby was coming in March. I am still working on living for the moment.

Never having had a girl, I cannot say how relationships come and go from their point of view. I certainly cannot remember that part of my growing up years in very much detail. Watching my sons and girls was interesting. One time I thought I would pray for an orphan girl for each of them as to not contend with her family. Fortunately, I matured in my thinking and simply prayed for God's best for each of them, and I realize today how thankful I am for my son's, their wives and families. At this point it was one down and one to go!

Jared met a girl in North Carolina at the church they were all attending. Darrell, Alisha and Jared had gotten involved in a church and once again made many new friends. They really cultivated their skills musically and sang often. This girl was a part of that period of time and sang with them, too. She travelled to Maryland several times and met the family. As a friend of Darrell and Alisha, she seemed to be fitting into our family. She was a good girl from a good family and things flowed along. Before Jared's second deployment, this time to Afghanistan, he quickly decided to propose to her. I was nervous about this whole new aspect of the relationship now that they were engaged and he was leaving. My son was a man. He had made life and death decisions in Iraq and I needed to allow him room to make this decision as well. By the time he came home from Afghanistan on his two week furlough, we all knew things were not good with this relationship, and we felt, as a family, the need to talk to Jared. Things had changed. We spent a day together as a family by going to the beach in Wilmington, NC and met up with Dustin. We shared our concerns and knew the final decision was up to Jared. Pushing too hard may push Jared away. The rest is history. Jared made the right decision, although it was a tough one. Today this girl is happily married to another military man and soon I will write about the girl that God had prepared all along for Jared.

Jared left for Afghanistan on January 19, 2007, just as Darrell was arriving home from Arizona. They missed seeing each other by a few minutes as Darrell tried to make it from the airport to Jared's departure point. Darrell saw Jared's bus pulling out as he arrived. Once again those same feelings surface...pride, fear, and anticipation. I was anxious for Jared to reach his destination, yet I knew on this deployment he would be spending most of his time flying missions, and I could only imagine where they would take him. Jared packed his guitar for this trip and I knew he would have a soothing piece of home with him. Now I was waiting again for the messages, phone calls, and letters, and listening intently when he called. I knew by hearing his voice that I would know if he was well, because that is what Moms do.

I sent Jared this verse: Psalm 121:7 NKJV "The LORD shall preserve you from all evil: he shall preserve your soul." Once again there were no promises that Jared would be safe from all harm, but I knew that God had him in His care and no matter what, all would be well. Later he told me of the comfort this verse brought, and even in the middle of gunfire with bullets whizzing past his head and helicopter, he knew God was there.

THE BIRTH OF OUR FIRST GRANDSON

In this life we have pain and trouble, but it is always interspersed with joy. I am thankful for the joy that always comes. This time it is coming in the form of our grandson! At this point in the story trumpets should sound.

On March 3rd, we received a phone call from Alisha. She and Darrell were in Home Depot and her water broke. Darrell being his cute self said he had to call for clean- up in aisle three. Michael and I had our bags packed to go to North Carolina and so did Alisha's parents. We had made so many trips down that road and knew the heavy traffic areas. Around Washington, DC was always interesting especially in the late afternoon. Really people…get out of our way! We arrived at the hospital that night and saw Alisha and Darrell. Michael and Dennis took up residence in the waiting room and I went back and forth checking on the progress while Dianna and Darrell stayed with Alisha. Everything was going forward, but it was a long night. I was trying to remain almost invisible, as this was our kids' event. Sometime in the early morning hours on the 4th, Dianna came running down the hallway. She said for everyone to come…Alisha wants all the parents in the room and this baby is coming! We did not expect this! Michael and Dennis were very sheepish as they entered the room and took their self assigned places above Alisha's head. I sat on the left side of Alisha and Dianna stood. I could not wait for this part to be over for Alisha. Suddenly, the baby was coming. I sat in awe as I watched our grandson unfold before my eyes. Never before had I experienced such an event and all I could do was cry. This completely unexpected honor will always be cherished. Aiden Michael Owens had entered this world. Darrell caught him and cradled him in his arms, and after cutting the cord, presented Aiden to his Mom. This is joy!

Aiden Michael Owens, this is my prayer for you. You are so sweet and kind, with such a big heart. I pray this follows you throughout your life. **Micah 6:8 NKJV "… What does the Lord require of you…to do justly, and to love mercy, and to walk humbly with your God?"**

We all left this little family alone and went to get some sleep. Dianna stayed for the next couple of weeks to help with all the new baby introductions. On the 23rd of March, Michael and I went back down and, as has happened so often over the years, Dianna and I acted as a tag team, and I stepped in for some special days with our new grandson. Pictures…how many pictures did we take? Trips…how many times did we go up and down the road? Sanford was close enough that we could make the trip in six and one half hours under the right conditions. Often, when I needed a "grandson fix", we would call to check with Alisha and their schedule, and we would hit the road. Alisha has never turned us down. My new role as "Nana" was more wonderful than ever imagined. Michael beams in his role as Granddaddy, too. God is good!

Life moved on. My thoughts were with Jared constantly as he was flying almost every day in Afghanistan. In May, Aiden, along with his parents made his first trip to Maryland. What fun to show off our grandson! We always looked forward to Darrell and Alisha's visits, but now it had changed. This was my opportunity to teach our grandson about his Nana and Granddaddy's house and all the fun we would have on McCauley Road. Now I realize we were carrying him around to "do" everything, but it was the beginning and we were planting images in his little mind of what we want to share with him and all others that follow. Pictures were constantly being taken! We also took many pictures of Aiden on the Owens' farm as things were progressing to sell. Hopefully, the pictures will place the farm in Aiden's memory.

Michael's life was very busy with the farm, our house and the family. So much for the empty nest...they may not live here anymore, but there is always action with family. We even managed another visit to Indiana to see my family and a visit to Chicago receiving the grand tour from Jim, Deneen and family. I always enjoy a big city trip, but I am always grateful to live in rural America.

We went back to North Carolina for some more grandson time. As grandparents, we could just go down and play with Aiden for a couple of days. Darrell would typically have some job for his Dad to accomplish, and Alisha and I would sneak in a shopping trip or two, but my main purpose was to play with Aiden. Of course, every trip to North Carolina meant taking something down for Darrell and Alisha. One trip the cabinet was so large that Michael had to put the spare tire on top of the Jeep. We really looked like country hicks on that trip. I think I prayed for Alisha to want something from Maryland just so we had a reason to go down. We did not really need an excuse, as Alisha always has welcomed us to their home. As Aiden grew, it was so fun when he would know who we were as we arrived and the greetings were wonderful. But with his growing the departures became more difficult, too. I always cried as we headed down the street to return home, but my heart was happy. Aiden is such a blessing, and I have often jokingly said he was my reward for not killing my son as a teenager.

August came and for the first time in many years I was not starting school. There were mixed emotions for me, but it was definitely time to move on. We began to attend Grace Bible Chapel and found many old friends and starting making some new ones. More change, but a change I needed that included a new circle.

In September, 2007, Jared came home for his two week furlough. We all met him at the airport in Raleigh, NC. Security, because of the USO, allowed us to go and be waiting at the gate when he came off the airplane. Alisha had a shirt made for Aiden that said, "Welcome Home Uncle Jared". This was the first time Jared was introduced to his nephew. People all around the airport were crying. Once again my heart was satisfied to touch my son again. The two weeks went by quickly and were slightly tainted by the story I told previously, but all ended well. We all spent some time in Maryland with grandparents and extended family with parties and pictures. On the 20th, Jared returned to Baghram for the final leg of his tour in Afghanistan, but not before Mom got a great big hug one more time.

Now one would think I would be satisfied and find plenty to keep me busy. But I needed something else to do. This restless streak has been a part of my life since I was a teenager. I needed something to focus my energy. In October, I attended orientation for substitute teachers in the county, and stepped out of my comfort zone into the public school arena again after many years in private school. I wanted to be in high school and chose North East High and Rising Sun High as the only two schools in which to substitute. It did not take long to find a real home in Rising Sun High School finding myself as busy as I wanted to be and often subbing every day of the week, but the schedule was my choice. We could still go to North Carolina when we wanted and take any other days off that I needed. I loved the staff and the students at RSHS and found satisfaction in my new job. A new circle of friends that also included some old friends!

Once again it was time for the holidays of 2007, and another year with one son missing. The bright spot was our first Christmas with a grandson. It was so fun having a little one around for Christmas morning and watch his excitement. Now you would think that I would remember all his gifts, but I just remember the fun in buying, wrapping, and seeing him open them. Christmas was never going to be the same now that grandchildren were here. Special memories!

January 16, 2008, took us to the Green Ramp again. Jared arrived home in the early morning hours with his unit and all the fanfare and excitement you can imagine. The pictures from this homecoming show us all, including Aiden in the stroller, and we were reunited again as a family. My son was home and in a few weeks he would be leaving the Army for civilian life again after giving six years of service. Jared was officially finished on April 25th and was going to take a well-deserved break before looking for a job. He had been trained well by the Army and knew helicopters. The Army is what you put into it, and Jared's hard work would pay off. Jared had worked toward a career and now had direction in his life.

January also meant the Owens farm was sold. The farm had been in the family since 1932 and so an era ended. The times spent there are sweet memories and we are thankful for those years and the family times there. The many family dinners over the years celebrating holidays or birthdays, the work days with Michael helping, and I would show up for lunchJ. My favorite times were watching the boys play with Grandmom and Granddaddy. Granddaddy even put up a basketball goal for his grandchildren. It was a great place for exploring and walking. Thanksgiving Day we had the tradition of going to the woods for crows' foot and we all used it to decorate for Christmas. It made great wreaths and bouquets. Target practice took place in the back yard. Then there was the pecan tree, walnut trees, the bonsai tree, and the sunflowers Pop Pop would grow. Great memories of the Owens Farm!

My Dad went into the hospital in Chicago for his NPH and I went to be with him for a few days. Darrell, Alisha and Aiden visited an injured friend at Walter Reed. Walter Reed hospital was a vivid reminder of the war, the cost in human lives and where my sons had been. Again, life continues on.

In April, Michael's mom moved into the apartment in Rising Sun and life changed again for her. She is such an example of being content. She keeps going with whatever life may hand her, and does it graciously. Mom Owens demonstrated an ability to adjust to changes and keep smiling as she moved on after the farm, taking with her great memories.

The second half of 2008 was full of activity and changes. The trips to North Carolina continued. Aiden turned one year old and we wanted to give him a swing set. Jared helped us by picking it up in his truck. We all went to Darrell and Alisha's and assembled the swing set. Aiden was such a big help as he carried off pieces. We enjoyed every part of our time there. Once the swing set was finished, it was time to push Aiden for hours and coax him to go down the slide. He immediately climbed up the ladder but was slow about coming down the slide. If Darrell, Alisha or Aiden needed us, we were there. So when Alisha called and Aiden was sick, I headed south to help out. I love my daughter-in-law to need me. Each trip allowed me to spend time with Aiden. I became his personal playmate and would not trade that for anything. He definitely has me wrapped around his finger and I enjoy it!

Jared took a trip with his childhood friend, Jeremy, to Puerto Rico for a few days after returning from Indiana to visit his grandparents and family. He was taking full advantage of time off after six years in the Army. I knew Jared was struggling with the aftermath of war, and he needed time away. Jared had missed his alone time, too, as that had always been important to him. My Mom eyes were careful to be aware of his struggles and to continue to pray specifically for my son.

Meanwhile, Michael retired from Aberdeen Proving Ground on June 27th after 30 years. But before retirement, he was able to take me for a ride on a Bradley Army vehicle, one of the many vehicles he had worked on over the years. I rode as a gunner and enjoyed riding around the track at Churchville Test Site. Michael was looking forward to retirement. We planned a trip to see my parents, sister and family and then on to Niagara Falls and a few days in Canada. This trip was just what we both needed. The past few years had taken more of a toll on us than I realized. We did it all at the falls…walking under the falls, riding the boat and staying in a beautiful hotel on the Canadian side looking over the falls. Montreal was a special treat with its French influences. I enjoyed watching Michael relish his days of doing whatever he wanted to do for a while. Life was easy for now, and all was well.

In June there was a graduation party for Brook Haines AND Jared met Julie. Steve Haines takes all the credit for bringing them together. They were amazing to watch. It boggles the mind when you think of all the places Jared had been and what he had done and how Julie had graduated from college and was beginning her career as a young adult when their paths crossed. Julie's Mom Mom will tell you she knew right away that they were "two peas in a pod", destined to be together. I liked Julie from the start. She is easy to be with and is a no frills girl. Julie and Jared were a perfect fit. By August, Jared was going on family vacation with the Moore's. God was once again putting our second son with a family that loves him as their own. David and Janice Moore, Jim, and the grandparents were to become Jared's family, too. In August, Jared interviewed for a job with Keystone and began working for them on August 18, 2008. This company would become Sikorsky Helicopter and Jared found his dream job building and flying helicopters. Julie is so comfortable to be around and she began to find a special place in my heart. Could I really be blessed with her as my next daughter-in-law? The best part for me was Jared would be living close enough to be able to spend time with him, since he now has a job in Coatesville and a girl in Calvert. My heart was very happy.

We were becoming more involved at Grace Bible Chapel. We attended regularly and joined a Bible study group. In this group we met a new bunch of people that would become dear friends as time progressed...a new circle. We met Theresa, Leica, Tom and Rhonda, Keith and Lorraine, and Dan and Cindy as cherished friends all through life group. Dave and Donna and Jack and Crystal are now some of our best friends and I cannot imagine life without them as they walked with us on our next incredible journey. I also participated in Apples of Gold, with Cindy, as a mentor for two sessions and enjoyed getting to know some wonderful young ladies and participate in a program that is dear to Cindy's heart. I was enjoying having Julie in and out of our house and getting to know her. Michael and I took several road trips in 2008, and we enjoyed his retirement together. I continued to substitute at RSHS and liked the flexibility of my schedule.

A strange incident happened one day while at the high school that resulted in a wonderful friendship. I saw someone who was substituting in another class that looked familiar, but I did not say anything. After coming home I went for a walk. While walking a car pulled into the driveway next door and that "someone" was driving. At that moment I realized it was my neighbor. We had only met once before, and I am ashamed to say I had not followed up on that first meeting. I took a chance that day and walked up the lane and knocked on the door. We both crammed much of our life stories into that afternoon conversation. Julie or "Neighbor Julie" as we often refer to her because of Jared's Julie, has become a dear friend. There is an obvious lesson to be learned here. When we are too busy to get to know our neighbor, then life has become TOO busy. When Mrs. Daly moved from the house next door I never thought about who would move in next or getting to know them. My indifference almost cost a friendship I would have never known. My life has been extra blessed by Faron and Julie.

Treasures can be so close. Be careful not to miss the obvious! Michael and I grew up in the same little town for several years and he was standing on the corner after his Army days and my running days. Remember Darrell's treasure in Alisha was just down the road. Jared's treasure in Julie, though they both had traveled far, was here also. My treasure in a friend was just next door. Look around for your next treasure could be right in front of you. Slow down and enjoy the trip and all those along the trail. You could be missing a special blessing... another circle.

Through the fall months, Jared was house hunting. In November, he found what he was looking for. He discovered an old house, very similar to our house that he grew up in, and decided to make the purchase. Several things came into play with this house. First of all, Julie approved and was willing to get dirty helping the renovation process go forward. Second, Michael would be put to work as much as he wanted. The hours were flexible and it was a labor of love for Jared. We all worked. We scrubbed, painted, ripped up carpet and even destroyed areas of the house making it livable. Julie, Janice, Betty, David, Ruthie, Donald, Darrell, Michael, and I did what we could to help Jared. We watched this old house convert into Jared's home. Jared was able to move into the house during renovations along with his cat, Stewart. The renovations took time and the results were worth it. We did not know right away, but there was a deadline. A wedding was going to happen in the near future. I must slow down as much will happen before the wedding takes place.

So much family time and none of which I take for granted. I am constantly thankful for time with husband, sons, wives, and grandchildren and circles of people in my life. None of us is promised tomorrow so do not ignore today!

The work on Jared's house continued. Julie was becoming a part of our family and Darrell and Alisha welcomed her with open arms. Family time was always welcomed and we were busy. One week Darrell had classes in Baltimore so Alisha and Aiden came up with him. Aiden spent the night with us one night while Alisha joined Darrell in Baltimore. The next day we went down and met them with plans to take Aiden to the aquarium for the day. When we parked the car Darrell and Alisha were there to meet us and Aiden started to cry. He thought his fun day to see the fish was ruined because Mom and Dad showed up, not realizing we were all going to see the fish.

My parents made a change this year also. They moved to Menomonee Falls, Wisconsin into an apartment. My little sister and her family would be moving there in the near future, also. Now they were farther away. In April we made a road trip to Indiana stopping at my sister's house. I always enjoy time with all those nieces and nephews. Then we went on to Wisconsin to visit my parents and see the new area. Mom and Dad seemed to be adjusting well to living in the apartment and were making new friends at their church before the Sikmas moved to the area. I was proud of their transition.

August 2009 saw us going down the road to North Carolina again. We arrived on a Thursday and as was typical we hit the ground running. Alisha ran downstairs with some clothes and asked me to change Aiden as we were getting ready to go out to dinner. I did not notice the camera in her hand as she returned standing on the stairs. The shirt I was putting on Aiden was printed with the words "I am the Big Brother". Sometimes I can be dense, as my family will attest, and it took a few seconds for it to sink in that another grandchild was on the way. Michael was watching and he, too, took a few moments to understand. Exciting days ahead as another March baby was coming. The next day we all went to Wilmington, North Carolina to visit Aunt Kay, Uncle Clarence, Dustin and Brandi. As usual it was a fun few days with our family, and the majority of my time was reading, playing, walking and talking with Aiden.

August 18, 2009, Jared prepared a special dinner at his house and during the evening proposed to Julie Anne Moore. We were so excited that she said yes and by the following June she would become Jared's wife. Now finishing the house was on the front burner. Julie also was free to participate more fully in the process, as it was to be her home, also. With Julie came her dog, Penny to join with Jared and Stewart. Julie was right for him and we all loved her very much. Wedding plans were being made and we had never seen Jared smile so much. It was so good to see my son happy! Once again my heart sings.

Time with friends was always interspersed in our busy days. Out to dinner with Cindy and Steve, Life Group meetings with our gang, girls' night out for me with ladies from school, a trip to NC, game time with Jared and Julie, and picnics with a campfire to roast marshmallows on those nice summer evenings were normal events of the summer and fall days. Out of town friends like the Roberts', Martins', and family from distant states would visit overnight or for a couple of days, and Darrell, Alisha and Aiden would come up the road for a visit. Life was good. For some reason, Candy and I started riding bikes this summer and fall. We would meet at the Conowingo Dam and ride the trails. Some days Andy and "neighbor" Julie would join us. We got serious, too, and thought we were doing well when our mileage for the week would total 60 + miles. We were in the best shape possible that fall and addicted to our bicycles. Michael liked to hike trails, so he and I would load up my bike, drive to a trail, and I would ride while he walked. I even tried kayaking with Andy and family during this fall.

I found this quote from Sir Arthur Conan Doyle in 1896 on a cycling blog: *"When the spirits are low, when the day appears dark, when work becomes monotonous, when hope hardly seems worth having, just mount a bicycle and go out for a spin down the road, without thought on anything but the ride you are taking."*

This is how I was feeling about my bicycle. I had found a good thing.

The guys were busy with their lives. Darrell was now on the 82nd Airborne Freefall Team and jumped many times each year at places such as local schools, college games, Fenway Park, NASCAR, festivals and Army celebrations. We were able to see him jump sometimes and enjoyed it all. A few times we were there when he carried in the United States Flag. It always brought such pride to watch him jump for the Army he had come to enjoy. I had come a long way since his first jump at Fort Benning, even though I was always glad to hear from him after the jumps were over. Jared was busy building helicopters, specifically the S-92, and then flying in them on their first flight. He was even flying over our house a couple of times! Flying here at home is far different from knowing he is flying in Afghanistan. I am proud of the work he does and glad to know he likes his job. He can talk for hours about his helicopters. There is joy in knowing my sons are happy. For having a Mom who was afraid of flying as a kid, my sons sure were spending much time in the air.

The holidays this year were filled with family. My parents flew in from Wisconsin and we had the entire crew for Thanksgiving dinner. It was an extra special year with Julie being added to the family soon as the wedding was being planned for June 2010 and having my parents visiting. So often I have talked about the holidays and how much I love them and all the family time that comes with both Thanksgiving and Christmas. All was well through Christmas. Michael gave me my FIRST NEW bicycle for Christmas, but he spoiled me and gave it early so I had some good riding days before winter. It was a Raleigh mountain bike. During the month of December we had 24 inches of snow, but I still got in a few rides before the end of January. But bigger things were on the horizon. Another grandson would be born in March and in June Jared and Julie would be married. Life was perfect...

Isaiah 55:8 KJV "For my thoughts are not your thoughts neither are your ways my ways, says the Lord."

The following are two of my favorite hymns over the years and these words were about to help carry me through another difficult time.

BE THOU MY VISION
Be thou my vision, O Lord of my heart,
Naught be all else to me, save that thou art.
Thou my best thought by day or by night
Waking or sleeping, thy presence my light.

Be thou my wisdom, and thou my true word

I ever with thee and thou with me, Lord.
Thou my great Father, I thy true son
Thou in me dwelling and I with thee one.

Riches I heed not, nor man's empty praise
Thou mine inheritance, now and always
Thou and thou only first in my heart,
High King of heaven, my treasure thou art.

High King of heaven, my victory won,
May I reach heaven's joys O bright heaven's Son!
Heart of my own heart, whatever befall,
Still be my vision, O Ruler of all.

(Mary Byrne 1905 Traditional Irish Melody)

COME THOU FOUNT OF EVERY BLESSING

Come, thou Fount of every blessing
Tune my heart to sing thy grace
Streams of mercy, never ceasing,
Call for songs of loudest praise.
Teach me some melodious sonnet
Sung by flaming tongues above,
Praise the Mount; I'm fixed upon it,
Mount of thy redeeming love.

O to grace how great a debtor,
Daily I'm constrained to be!
Let thy grace, Lord, like a fetter,
Bind my wondering heart to thee.
Prone to wonder, Lord I feel it,

Prone to leave the God I love.
Here's my heart, Lord, take and seal it.
Seal it for thy courts above.

(Robert Robinson 1758)
Public Domain

Chapter 8

JOURNEY WITH CANCER*

(*) *Remember this is my journey and my perspective and nothing written here should be taken as medical advice. The protocol followed was designed for me.*

I read one time that changing direction in life is not tragic, but losing the passion for life is. My direction was changing! My love for life was not...life is worth the fight! I was passionate about hanging around to watch my grandsons grow and to dance with my son on his wedding day, but the list did not end there. I wanted to grow old with Michael, and 57 was not old, and was hoping to be around to see more grandchildren as a result of Jared and Julie's marriage.

January/February 2010 were unusually cold and snowy months. After having had a 24" snowfall in December no one expected more very large snowfalls in January/February. Jared was here to help shovel snow with his Dad and it seemed there was no end to the snow. I would venture out to help but quickly would become exhausted. During the following days walking up the steps became a struggle. I simply thought that not riding my bicycle as often had taken a toll and I was getting out of shape quickly.

Finally, in February it was time for a routine blood test. One Wednesday I went into Rising Sun for my blood draw as usual. That evening my doctor called telling me to come to Christiana Hospital the following morning for a blood transfusion as my hemoglobin was 6.5. If I had any chest pain, I was not to wait until morning, but come immediately. One answer...my low count was the reason I was so tired.

Now we had another question…why? We were sent to Dr. Hosford, an oncologist/hematologist. We both liked her from the start, but this is not a doctor you want to visit. So began the cycle of blood work, type and cross, transfusion, blood work, type and cross, transfusion…two units each transfusion.

Now you may notice I keep changing the pronouns. Sometimes it is me and sometimes it is we, although Michael is in this with me for the long haul. As I write this down, his active involvement will be evident. Most of the time it is we, but when I am the one being stuck it is all me. Needles are not my favorite thing, and I do wish we could take turns or something.

The Birth of our Second Grandson

Now life is continuing to go on and it is time for those trumpets to sound once again! Alisha and Darrell were still living in North Carolina and grandson number two was coming soon. On Monday, March 29th, Darrell called to say that Alisha was sick and asked if we could come now to help with Aiden. We were already packed as we knew the baby could come at any time so we were on the road very quickly that day heading south. We were enjoying the ride and looking forward to what was coming when the phone rang again. This time Darrell said they were on their way to the hospital as things were getting started. Suddenly our mood changed. Get out of the way you crazy drivers we have a grandson arriving soon! When Darrell called, we were just south of Washington, DC in heavy traffic. We arrived at the hospital around 9:00 PM, saw Darrell and Alisha, and we knew the baby would be here soon. Dianna and Dennis could not come right away so another good friend was already there with Alisha and she and Darrell were coaching her through. You see as mom-in-law I know my place and I took it off to the side as the action began. Michael again was standing at Alisha's head and he rubbed her shoulder. Darrell was ready to assist when the baby came. At 10:25 PM Eli Jaxson Owens was born! Such a sweetie and Mom and baby were doing well. Once again I was honored to be there for his birth. Two grandsons… We stayed until the weekend to help out with Aiden and Eli. I enjoyed helping Alisha and Darrell with anything I could. My stamina was low and at this point none of us knew how sick I really was. Michael and I took Aiden out for a special day on Friday to downtown Fayetteville. We went to the train station to watch the trains and had lunch outdoors at a café along the street. We visited the Airborne Museum and every soldier was "daddy". It was a special day with Aiden. Dianna and Dennis arrived on Saturday and we exchanged places once again. We knew we had enjoyed the moment this time and now must prepare as best we could for what was ahead.

Eli Jaxson Owens this is my prayer for you. Since you are our trusting and fearless one I pray that you learn to fear only the Lord and trust Him. **Psalm 112:1 NKJV "...blessed is the man that fears the Lord, who delights greatly in his commandments."**

Another life changing event was occurring at the same time. Charlotte's fiancée, Butch was dying with leukemia. We had visited him for the last time on Sunday before we left for North Carolina on Monday and he passed away 20 minutes before Eli was born. The cycle of life was very evident that day.

On April 8th, Dr. Hosford did my first bone marrow biopsy. No details about the procedure from me as I survived and Michael was by my side. The doctor started Procrit shots. Procrit is a growth factor for red blood cells. Procrit and transfusions were given regularly as we waited for the results of the biopsy to come back. We learned to give the Procrit shots at home. Going to the pharmacy to pick up the prescription of Procrit was traumatic. Neighbor Julie had taken me to the pharmacy and the pharmacist wanted to see me. You see this prescription was very expensive. When she told me how much, I was very upset. I replied, "It would be cheaper to die." She and my friend made me promise never to say that again. The realization of our growing medical bills began to sink in and we were thankful for good insurance.

On April 22nd we met with Dr. Hosford and heard the diagnosis of Myelodysplasia Syndrome. A quick explanation is that the blood cells made of red cells, white cells, and platelets were dying once they left the marrow. MDS, as I will refer to it from now on, were scary words from the doctor on this day. Our next question...now what? For now it was more of the same with blood work, type and cross, and another transfusion. I was so excited for more needles.

Now Dr. Hosford made an appointment for us at Johns Hopkins Hospital to see Dr. B. Douglas Smith whose expertise is MDS. May 3rd was to be our first trip to Hopkins. Before we went to Hopkins we saw Dr. Weidner, our family doctor, to make sure he was in the loop.

The journey into the unknown was about to begin and a much unexpected circle was about to form. Storms and their paths are often unpredictable, and I fought to remain in the eye.

I will never forget the first time I walked into the Kimmel Cancer Center at Johns Hopkins. This massive foyer of people and the first thing I noticed was it was full of sick people, and I did not feel sick. People were walking around with bald heads and IV poles and little did I realize that one day soon I would be one of them. It was all very overwhelming. How thankful I was for Michael being at my side.

More lab work was on the schedule after the registration, and then in to see Dr. Smith. At least we had a doctor whose name we could pronounce, as some of the names at Hopkins were unusual. He was the kindest man, who put us at ease immediately, and he spoke with such confidence helping us both to know we were not alone. He explained in detail the disease and gave us the prognosis. After learning that Chromosome 7 was 45% missing, he told us that all I had was two years without treatment. Now that was a shock. He also explained what treatment I needed. By now the addition of AML (Acute Myelogenous Leukemia) was added to the diagnosis. The only chance for a cure, because of that missing Chromosome, was a bone marrow transplant. The steps to the transplant would begin now. Dr. Smith (or Best, Doug, as he always signs our emails and we affectionately call him) and his nurse practitioner, Valerie Ironside, became very dear people to us.

Slow down everyone. We had a new grandson that arrived in March and our son's wedding will be in June. I already knew that I did not want to begin any chemotherapy until after the wedding, if at all possible. I had a son to dance with on June 18th. Telling our family the details of what was ahead was difficult. Talking to our sons and wife/ fiancé was the second time I cried. Truth was there was no time for tears or wasted energy. I had cancer to beat! I sound tough, but I had many weak moments. It was time to start the plan.

By the end of May my sisters were sent a kit to see if they were a match. Lynn's kit was sent to Germany and Deneen's kit was sent to Wisconsin. I had a 25% chance of a sibling being a full match. Waiting...

From Lynn:

Isaiah 43:1 NKJV "I have called you by your name; you are mine."

19 "...I will even make a road in the wilderness, and rivers in the desert."

From Deneen:

"Difficulty is the very atmosphere of a miracle...it is a miracle in its first stage."

"The clinging hand of His child makes a desperate situation a delight to Him."

These quotes taken from Streams in the Desert by Mrs. Charles E Cowman, Zondervan Press, 1996.

More of the same...labs, transfusions, Procrit and then do it all again. Also the doctors wanted me to have a dental check-up and a CT of the sinuses. Things were lining up for the transplant when the time was right.

Trying to live a normal life when you are headed to the biggest fight of your life is difficult. Darrell, Alisha and the boys came to Maryland. Darrell was to jump with his 82nd Airborne Team into the Preakness and he had gotten some VIP passes. Jared and Julie, Susie, Jason and Liz and Michael and I were going to the Preakness. It ended up that the wind was too high for a safe jump. We were all disappointed, but still enjoyed our day at the Preakness with several horse races and many people to watch.

June was here! Life was anything but normal. Michael began to have some problems with his eye and on the 4th had eye surgery and was home for the couch for one week. Jared's house needed the main bathroom finished before the wedding. When Michael's week was over he was back to work at Jared's and they finished on June 14th. So now all is progressing again. Even though we may never understand the full plan on this side of heaven, God was active in the lives of my family.

Both of my sisters were very willing to do whatever was needed, and we waited on the results. My youngest sister, Deneen, had given birth to her eleventh child on April 24, 2010. Little Phillip was a Trisomy 18 baby. Yet through all of this she remained willing to be my donor if she proved to be a match. Once again, God demonstrated his control. Philip was a blessing for his 61 days here on earth. I never met this nephew, but heard the stories and saw pictures day to day of the little triumphs along the way. Never was a little boy given so much love in such a short time. With a house full of siblings and loving parents and grandparents, he was cuddled and loved every day of his life until on June 24, 2010, he went to be cradled in the arms of Jesus. Life is full of unforeseen twist for us all. In the middle of it all God knew the next steps. He knew this when we were all kids running around carefree. It is even more amazing that God knew before the foundation of the world. Without the knowledge of God's complete control, my life would have crumbled. In June, we learned that my sister, Lynn, was a full match or perfect match as she prefers to call herself.

There was still much preparation to take place before the transplant and more than a few logistics to work out since Lynn lived in Germany. We both had much testing to go through to be sure we were ready before the big day. Blood transfusions kept me going for now.

First there was a wedding to not only attend, but enjoy!

Jared's Army buddies, Brandon and Tommy were coming to be in his wedding. Darrell, Alisha and boys arrived, too! Things were coming together. On Thursday, the guys all went groundhog hunting and came home with eight groundhogs. It made a great picture with the groundhogs draped over the rock surrounded by all the fearless hunters. Rehearsal dinner went well on Friday. We had it catered and used the tent that was set up in the Moore's backyard for the wedding the next day. Julie had always dreamed of having her wedding reception in the backyard. Rehearsal was entertaining to watch as Jared and Julie were enjoying their moment! Jared and Brandon entertained us that night with guitar and accordion like they had played together in Afghanistan. I enjoyed watching my sons interact that day, and it was extra special to have Darrell sing and play his guitar at his brother's wedding and watch Aiden walk down the aisle as Uncle Jared's ring bearer.

Julie was a beautiful smiling bride, her strawberry blonde hair gleaming, and my pleasure was watching Jared as his bride is walked down the aisle by her father. They had all four of us parents stand with them and acknowledge our approval of this union. Somehow on this day I was focused on the wedding and all it entailed and did not even think about my fight ahead. My early childhood friend, Chris Gambill Bradfield, played the organ for their wedding, Darrell handled the song with ease and our oldest grandson walked down the aisle without hesitation. The reception was relaxed and enjoyable. My wish came true as I danced with Jared to a special song. He and I talked, and I told him how proud of him I was and how thankful I was for Julie coming into his life and he told me he was proud of me as his Mom. God had the perfect girl all picked out for Jared! As I watched them drive away to catch a boat for their honeymoon cruise, all I could say was "Thank you, Lord"!

...back to the fight. On June 28th I began my chemotherapy. We started with Vidaza shots...three needles everyday for a week, a three week break and then start again. Now the purpose of the chemotherapy was actually to make me as strong as possible before transplant by destroying as many cancer cells as possible. This routine was followed for several weeks through Dr. Hosford's office. The shots were painful, and they left my skin very irritated as the nurse always looked for new spots to stick. Special people such as Beth, Terri and Shirley came into my life during treatment at Union Hospital.

Finally, after another office visit in September with Dr. Smith, we tentatively set a date. A few more days of finalizing and the phone came that everything was a go. By the end of October the decision was made that I would be admitted to the hospital and preparing for one of the biggest days of my life. Protocol differs from patient to patient. Some transplants are done on an outpatient status with going to the hospital daily, while others, like me, are admitted to 5B until the counts begin to rise again and then become outpatient on a daily basis.

Lynn arrived from Germany on October 12th. She hit the ground running. We both had much testing to do that week and I had another bone marrow biopsy. All was coming together so we all knew the timing was right. Now was the time! Heart scan, more blood work, CT scans and a BMT class. Lynn and I compared notes to see who gave the most vials of blood that week. I met with Valerie and Lynn met with Mindy. We had separate teams to keep it all impartial. We had a tour of the unit, met more people, had more consults and signed more papers. We were told from the start not to look around at others as each of us would be different. All was a go!

Before the big event started, some friends got together to hold a fundraiser to help with the expenses of the trips back and forth to Hopkins for Michael and finding an apartment for the month after I was released as we needed to stay close. I was reminded of the four friends that brought their friend to Jesus to be healed and went to all the trouble of lowering him through the roof because of the crowd. My friends, Cindy, Julie, Andy, and Candy were willing to do whatever it took to help us through this time. The event was to be a Run, Walk, Hike, or Bike day at Nottingham Park. Many others helped on that day including my family and a teacher from RSHS and her husband. They had T-shirts made for the event. Alisha along with Aiden and Eli helped with the front design on the shirt and had kept it all a secret. The shirt read "BRING IT FOR NANA" with the footprints of those two grandsons underneath. Event day was overwhelming as people came and participated and gave. They also had found some corporate sponsors and even some strangers drove into the park that day and donated for the cause. My sister, Lynn, and I were able to be there even though the wearing of the mask to protect me had already started. The generosity of that day and many other gifts paid our expenses through the next two month journey we were about to encounter. It was almost down to the penny that our out-of-pocket costs were covered. Our all knowing God is incredible. One person gave a sizable amount in response to someone giving him a sizable amount when they needed it for their son. They attached a note telling us that perhaps one day we would have the same opportunity. People at church gave with generous hearts; the church gave as well as the generosity of RSHS which gave Visa Cards for gas and other expenses. We were truly awestruck by the love demonstrated toward us.

A few days before I went into the hospital, Pastor Steve, Pastor Wayne, and two elders came to the house to pray with us. Pastor Steve anointed me with oil and they asked God to bring glory to Himself through the coming days.

The following Sunday would be our last time to attend Grace before entering the hospital. Because of the need to be cautious, we would arrive to the service about 10 minutes late and I was wearing that mask. When we walked into the auditorium that morning it took a couple of seconds to begin to realize what was happening. Everyone on the platform was wearing one of the fundraiser shirts and then we realized that a large portion of the congregation was wearing one also. Pastor Steve even wore the shirt! Such love and support was shared by a group of people that day and we knew we were and would be prayed for through the coming days. An encouragement I will never forget.

Now for entering the hospital, I thought I was prepared. My parents and sisters and families had given me a little HP Notebook to take with me along with my cell phone. Jared put some of my favorite songs on the computer. One of my favorites was "How Can I Keep From Singing His Praise" by Chris Tomlin which I hummed often throughout my stay. I was so thankful for the ways to keep in touch with my family and friends on a daily basis if I felt like communicating. Plus, I could receive all the encouraging emails that began to pour in from the first day on, or put on my earphones and listen to music.

We woke up early this morning as we needed to be at the hospital by 7 a.m. Bags were packed and ready for this adventure...this new beginning. I knew leaving home that morning would be difficult, but God had a very simple plan. It was dark and foggy and as we went to leave, yet I noticed a spider web running from the roof of the house to the Jeep. I commented that it was long enough to be a zip line and we laughed at the comparison to the journey ahead. Simple details…never doubt that God is in them.

Day one in Johns Hopkins was October 28, 2010. There was no time to be afraid as the activities were endless and the staff was trained at putting patients at ease. The first event was inserting a Hickman catheter in my chest. A young doctor walked in to begin the procedure and he looked about the age of my oldest son. He talked and laughed with me and quickly put me at ease. Actually that was not too bad. Michael and I got settled into my room. The unit has a pressurized filtered air system as a first stop for germs entering the unit, so as you enter the doors are suctioned closed. I had to smile and said it was a step up for only what I imagine is the clanging sound made when prison doors are slammed. I never doubted that I would walk out of that hospital one day, although many trying days were to come. The staff was wonderful. Our dear friends, Cindy and Steve, came down for the day to encourage us on in getting this process started and they continued to visit often.

It was a comfortable room with a huge window, but the view was not the greatest. A chair in the corner provided the best view as I could see between the two tall buildings, open skies, and if it was clear I could even see a tree in the distance. I soon learned that if I were alert I could watch the helicopters come and go from the hospital. That sight made me realize that many others were in pain and facing a crisis beyond my own. The only comfort in hearing helicopters was the reminder of my son. From that day on I was determined to find something new out that window even if it was only a brick formation never noticed before. One of my nephews, Andrew, made a beautiful poster that we had framed and brought to the hospital and hung it on the wall. The Parkes, going through similar circumstances, had shared this verse with me. Andrew made the poster, and I from then on carried that verse as my own.

Psalm 57:1 NKJV "Be merciful to me, O God, be merciful to me! For my soul trusts in you, in the shadow of your wings will I make my refuge until these calamities have passed by."

Bone Marrow Transplant

No time was wasted as the chemotherapy began on the same day as admittance. We all hear the awful stories of chemo and know it is a poison they are running into my veins. I was apprehensive, but relaxed in knowing God's control and so many prayers. For the next three days they filled me with Busulfan with Dilantin for a total of 16 units. I also had a new best friend. The bags filled with chemo ran through the IV machine to my Hickman. It was not long until I realized when getting out of bed to head to the bathroom you must pull that machine with you. So as a result of my new close relationship, the machine was named. Everybody (thing) needs a name and this was Fred. Fred and I spent many days together and we learned to dance nicely. Wearing my mask became routine.

During this time I received many phone calls, cards and emails. Darrell, Alisha, and Aiden made the trip from home as they had been visiting, helped with the fundraiser and spent time with us before I went into the hospital. I had worn that mask for a few weeks now and Aiden and Eli seemed not to mind. Then they visited at Hopkins. Eli was just a baby so he stayed with his Granny, but Aiden was old enough to know a little of what was happening and was allowed to visit me for a few minutes. At this point I could still leave the unit, wearing my mask and pushing Fred, and we made our way to the main lobby of the old Johns Hopkins building. I had become one of those sick people pushing a pole that I noticed on that first visit. Aiden and I enjoyed visiting the large statue of Jesus and we posed for a picture. We followed them down the hall and said our goodbyes. My heart needed the boost. They stayed a couple more days and stopped in as a family before heading back to North Carolina. On this stop, Eli came to the lobby on my floor. Not being allowed to hold and snuggle him was difficult, but I was grateful to see them all one more time. The next time we would be together would be when I was released to the apartment. The goodbyes that day were etched in my mind for the coming weeks. The sweet memories, my photo book and the digital picture frame that Darrell and Alisha had given me would have to suffice for now.

Meanwhile, my sister, Lynn, took off in an airplane to visit our parents, sister and family, her children and grandchildren for a few days. People were shocked. After all, was not I afraid something would happen to her or she would get sick or whatever else the mind could imagine. Somehow I knew that God had not brought us this far without seeing it completed and ultimately the details were up to Him.

The critical time was coming, but first they needed to destroy all my bone marrow. On November, 1, 2010, the multiple doses of Cytoxan with Mesna were started. Once my marrow was destroyed, the insertion of my sister's marrow was essential. The good news is my sister came back!

I cannot overlook a story from one of the doctors on my team. Bone marrow transplants were first tried in the sixties and most failed. The research has been intense over the years and BMT's have become successful. This doctor told us that in the early sixties when the drug Cytoxan first came into existence, it was experimented with on sheep. One of the known side affects was hair loss so someone had the great idea to shear sheep an easier way. The experiment worked, but all the sheep died. I must admit he made me laugh and I always enjoy a good story. Another reason to be thankful for continued cancer research. The patients now have a chance of life, but one does lose all the hair.

During this time of preparing, and after a visit from the social worker, I decided to attend the support group meeting that week. Now we were told everybody's story is different so do not plan to follow the same time schedule of other patients you meet. Capacity for BMT patients on the unit is seventeen and for many reasons many do not or cannot attend. This day I met several others in various stages of the transplant process. Three of us were waiting and two of us would have transplant on the same day while others in the group were post-transplant. One meeting is someone I will remember the rest of my days. I met a very special person in Ann Myers whose room was right next door. I was taken by her spirit and determination immediately. Ann and I were bound together by our circumstances and her story will always be a part of my story. Her donor was her brother. If you ever talk about donors, I guarantee tears will flow as we remember such an act of love offered by a family member or a stranger. I also met Ann's family, her Mom, her husband, Jon and her two sons, Emory and Joseph. Through our process, Ann and I walked the halls together often as we updated each other on our individual journeys. If Ann or I was having a bad day, her Mom, Gretchen, and Michael would keep each other informed. Sometimes people physically become a part of your life for only a moment, yet the bond is forever.

On November 2, 2010, the chemotherapy was complete, but not without much physical distress. Hopkins then allowed my body two days of rest. Encouragement came in the form of many visitors such as Andy, Lynn, Michael, and Julie and Faron. My blood counts are dropping and finally the day of transplant is here. Transfusions of red cells and platelets were required and my white count hit zero.

At Hopkins this day, Day Zero is known as your new birthday and a celebration is in order. Everyone celebrates your new birthday as your family and friends are encouraged to join the celebration. My type of transplant is an allogeneic bone marrow transplant. There are several types of transplants and some different ways to harvest the marrow and the rich stem cells found in the bone marrow. Dr. Smith and his team had made all the decisions on the approach to be taken in my best interest. So, on the morning of November 5, Lynn was admitted to the surgical unit and ready to begin the harvest of her cells. The marrow would be taken from her hips ultimately leaving her very black and blue. Her surgery began around 9:30 a.m. Michael was there with her for the beginning and then stayed outside the surgical unit most of the day. In my room the excitement was building. My nurse was very excited and explained in detail what I should expect. Our son, Jared, was able to take the day off and stayed with me for the day. Michael came to check on me a few times, but stayed close to Lynn. Around 4:00 we knew Lynn's procedure was over. She had given around two liters of bone marrow for me. Cindy and Steve were present and Andy showed up with a "birthday cake". Now I could not handle eating, but sure enjoyed the party for my chance at life. Around 4:30 p.m. that precious marrow was brought into my room. They had prepared a sling to hold the bag safely and began running the marrow straight into my Hickman bypassing Fred to preserve all those fragile cells.

My nurse, Zack, stayed with me through the entire process. No words can describe this event and all the significance it held. Lynn had given me the gift of life. The life giving marrow ran into my blood stream until 7:30 p.m. The nursing staff told us they cannot explain how that marrow knows where to go. They rightly choose to call it a miracle. Finally, at 8:30 p.m. in came the person I had been longing to see. An attendant wheeled Lynn into my room, and all we could do was embrace and cry. The gift was given and now the receiver needed to do the rest.

The next two days were days of rest. Michael had taken Lynn to our house that night to get some much needed rest, given her some pain meds the doctor had prescribed and she rested through her first night. The next morning Lynn had her post-op check and was released. She and Michael came into my room and spent a few hours. Lynn was sore and tired, but overall doing well. She always tells me someday I will hear the full story of how she really felt after her donation of marrow. The problem with telling me later is that her story will have grown way out of proportion. Two days after transplant Lynn was ready to fly back to Germany. The airline had promised to take good care of her on the flight as she even carried a letter from Hopkins telling what she had done. The airline did not keep their word, but God always keeps His. Our friend, Eleanor had taken Lynn to the airport and it became apparent that any promises made by the airline would be broken. Our God of details had it already worked out. A couple that Lynn had actually met before in Germany were on the same flight and upon hearing the situation promised Eleanor that they would take good care of her all the way back to Dennis. As it turned out that couple was even seated directly behind her on the airplane, helped her through customs, and saw her to the arms of her waiting husband. It would take her body about two weeks to replace the marrow and she slowly recovered from the painful hip. I am forever grateful.

During these two days of rest I said goodbye to my sister and began the wait. Day 2 was a Sunday. The day seemed long. The Ravens were playing football at home that day so I tried to focus on the game. After the game, Faron came to visit. Michael was at my side. Candy and family came to visit. Andy stopped in for a little while as she was leaving on vacation for the next two weeks. The phone rang and it was Darrell and Alisha. Aiden wanted to talk to me. Just hearing his voice was a boost, but his words were such a sweet reminder. He said, "Nana, Jesus is taking care of you." I needed that! Darrell told me that Aiden prayed for me faithfully and Alisha said he told others that his "Nana was sick and in the hospital". All the way to this point I had not begged God for healing, but on this day I did tell Him I sure would like to see my grandchildren grow up.

Now I was receiving more chemotherapy. A cocktail of Cytoxan with Mesna, Benadryl and dexamethazone was given for two more days. Marlene visited on this second day of chemo and I only remember because I wrote it in my journal. By day five and at a low point physically, my family and friends continued to be a comfort. Now I was confined to the unit. The trip to Baltimore for family and friends was not an easy one and parking was expensive, but still they came. Jack and Crystal, Jared and Julie, Alisha, Darrell and grandsons, Mom O, Jared's Pastor Mike, Darrell and Alisha's friend Jeff Geyer, Candy and family, Susie, Ruth Wilson, Marlene, Keith our neighbors and many others that are mentioned throughout the story came. Some of the visitors were expected and others much unexpected. I was so grateful for each one.

November 10-15 are blurred with a mixture of good and bad days. I was sick with nausea, vomiting, diarrhea and very weak. The number of nausea pills available is amazing and they searched for one that worked. Hydration was important and my weight was monitored carefully. My hair, though I had it cut short before being admitted, was falling out rapidly so a lady came up and completely shaved my head and I did not even care. My white counts had dropped to zero which had been the goal. I was given more platelets and red cells. Those days before transplant and through the first chemotherapy I had walked to the exercise room and rode the stationery bike for ten minutes each morning. Now it was all I could do to get out of bed. My goal from the start had been to be up, showered, dressed and sitting in my chair by the time the first rounds were made. For now this goal was difficult. This was the time of waiting. Each morning as the group of doctors paraded into my room I listened carefully to every word. These were the days when I was most tested. The big question every morning was, "are my white blood counts starting their rise". Each night the nurse would take blood from my Hickman and each morning my nurse would write the numbers on a chart hanging on the outside of my bathroom door. The platelets and red cells began to grow and I required fewer transfusions. The white count was the one for which we all held our breath and waited to begin growing.

Since each nurse had two patients, we spent much time with our nurses and each had a story to tell. They were our caregivers, but more than that they were our greatest encouragers. Many of them had worked in the BMT unit for a long time and seen the great progress made in the success of transplants. Trisha was one of those with much experience in the unit, but ultimately Pete became my favorite as he could make the best Ensure and chocolate ice cream shake. Every doctor, nurse, assistant and service staff gave of themselves to see me through this journey. The only food I despised was a banana. One day when the snack guy came through and I chose a banana, only to lose it immediately. For months, even the smell of a banana made me nauseous. The quality of care was excellent.

Dr. Smith told me from the start that I would settle into the rhythm of the unit and it was happening. Mornings with the rounds could be counted on as they fell consistently in the same time frame. My own routine of showering, dressing, doing some stretches in bed, sitting in my chair and reading my Bible, looking out the window for something new while listening to music on my computer and taking my first walk of the day around the unit became a ritual. The walking was greatly encouraged. By the time my morning routine was over, Michael would arrive, catching me up on the latest news and bringing in fresh laundry. Before you knew it lunch arrived. The guys who brought the meals were compassionate and caring always meeting every request possible as we all fought nausea. After lunch we would take a walk again and soon Michael was off in his search for a meal. Thursday brought our support group meetings with Lacey and time with others. Michael stays through dinner and between seven and eight o'clock, he heads home. Before he leaves he help me get ready for the night and often leaves me sitting in my chair. My evenings are spent reading emails, writing a new update to friends and family and sometimes an unexpected visitor will appear breaking up the evening. Since focusing is hard for any period of time, reading is in short spurts and following the story line of a TV show is impossible. The evening includes those blood draws then lights out and hopefully sleep well to begin it all again tomorrow.

There is an older building in my line of sight and one day I asked Michael if he could identify the building. I learned that it was Reed Hall and Michael had stayed in that building long ago when he was dating a nurse. This was a new story to me and reminded me how glad I am to be the one who snagged him! My careful observation out my window had given some new information today.

If I was having a good day, Fred and I would make our way to the exercise bike for five or ten minutes. Day 9 was a Sunday, and the doctors all thought my progress was good. Doctors said this morning that some people go through this without ever having a fever. I dared to hope that would be true. Michael came a little later today, arriving after church. Candy, Gary and girls, along with Susie, appeared as well as Cindy and Steve. This was my first day to show off my beautiful bald head. Many phones call came in that afternoon and the Sunday passed quickly. Not all days went so well, and I did not take this one for granted. That same feeling seem to overwhelm me each morning as I waited for the counts to rise. Jared had put some music on my computer and donning the headset seemed to always calm my anxious heart. Jared had also sent me the same verse I sent to him in Afghanistan because it brought him comfort. I focused on Psalm 121:7 once again. I was at peace in the eye of this storm and what God chose was fine with me.

I was so thankful for my little notebook computer and sent emails on a regular basis to my friends and family. The following are some of those excerpts of emails sent from the hospital, apartment and finally home.

Day 1

"...the events of yesterday reminded me of Jesus Christ as my "donor" whose coming rescued me and gave me eternal life. What my sister has done for me is truly Christ-like."

Day 35

"...greeted today with the doctor saying he had great news for us. The recent blood tests showed I now have 100% of Lynn's cells. Needless to say I began to cry, as this is so incredibly fast. Prayers have been answered again today. Thanks for praying and please do not stop."

Day 90

"...I wanted to tell you that hair is overrated. After all, only the follicles on your head are alive and the rest is dead. Yes, I continue to be bald, but bald has its advantages. When I roll out of bed nothing is sticking up in all directions from my head. I am using the same bottle of baby shampoo I bought before entering the hospital, no hair products needed or salon appointments, so cost are greatly reduced. Now before you shave your head, remember not every head looks good bald."

People and the little things they do are so important. We have learned some of the dos and don'ts of helping others through our experience. I hope I always remember some of these lessons. Probably the biggest lesson is seeing that a person with a true heart of giving gives without asking. For example, when someone calls and says "What can I do?" unless they are family we probably will not give them a list. The greatest was when someone called and said "I am making dinner for you tonight, ok?" or, "I am coming to clean." One of many instances was the neighbor who fixed dinner for Michael, put it in the refrigerator, and turned on lights for him. So many showed up with food for Michael as his days were long and his nights were short.

Day 11 brought a fever of 38 C. Usually that is not a big deal, but in my case it could mean the start of a life threatening infection. So the medical team goes into action. Blood cultures, chest x-ray and antibiotics are done immediately. When the cultures grew we learned there was a blood infection and the antibiotic was changed to fit the infection. Receiving platelets and red cells was a continual need. There were very small improvements in my white blood count and I would ask the doctors if it was time to celebrate yet. The answer would be "Not yet." Finally on Day 15 my WBC made a move. The numbers went from 160-420. Now when the doctors came in I asked if I could be excited yet. They replied, "NOW." Over the next few days my numbers began to multiply rapidly. The increasing white count, neutrophils and platelet count meant the new marrow was beginning to form. This was cause for celebration! The miracle was happening and my body was making new bone marrow. The next step in my progress would be moving from the hospital to an apartment. I could not wait.

On Day 17 Michael worked to secure an apartment. Johns Hopkins helped us by supplying a list of places suitable to rent. We did not want to rent too soon because of the cost, but now Michael walks into the hospital being told to find a place as I will be released soon. The choices narrowed because we needed it now. The apartments beside the hospital would not allow children to visit and seeing those grandchildren was a requirement! After several phone calls Michael found one place available and said yes, sight unseen. My only request had been an apartment with a view. And always being the one to complicate things, I spiked another fever. Actually that gave an extra day or two for Jared and Julie to help Michael move a few things to the furnished apartment and wipe it down in preparation for me. Also, Julie came to the hospital to learn how to take care of my Hickman.

Darrell, Alisha and the boys were up from North Carolina and the plan was to come and spend Thanksgiving Day with me. When they arrived at the hospital, Pete came in my room and said I was being released. Day 21 and I was out of there in a whirlwind. Alisha packed my bag and I seemed to move quickly, since I had this fear someone would change their mind. Off to the apartment with Jared, Julie, Darrell, Alisha, Aiden, Eli, Susie, Michael and me. When Michael took me upstairs and unlocked the door, I could not believe my eyes. If you ever doubted that God cares about the little things, you should have stood in that doorway with me. The view was spectacular with windows from floor to ceiling in the living room/dining/kitchen and in the bedroom. It was overlooking Camden Yards and the Inner Harbor. We were living on the fifteenth floor of the Zenith Apartments on Pratt Street. One could not have ordered anything more. One little detail…it was Thanksgiving Day with an apartment full of people and very little food. Michael and Darrell went on a very long walk, finally finding an open Subway and brought back subs. I had peanut butter and crackers. It was the BEST Thanksgiving ever. One of the first things I asked my family to do was to rearrange the furniture. I think I was on my way back!

Now was time for a new routine in the apartment. At first I felt insecure after the excitement of Thanksgiving, because I seemed so far away from Hopkins. In reality we were about 10 minutes from parking garage to parking garage. No more constant checks from the staff as we were on our own. My temperature had to be monitored constantly and any number over 38 Celsius meant a return trip to Hopkins until the cause was determined. No Tylenol meant no cheating. Now we would take a daily trip to the hospital to Inpatient/Outpatient Care Continuum now referred to as IPOP. Daily at IPOP they would take blood through the Hickman and soon it was determined what my body needed. The only additions in oral prescriptions to my daily regime were Valtrex and Dapsone. One was to protect from viruses and the other to protect my skin. Infection and Graft versus Host disease (GVHD) were now my greatest enemies. Two days in the apartment and we were headed back to the hospital with a temperature. Blood cultures, x-ray, ct, two units of platelets and two units of red cells were required that night. I was admitted back into my old room. Discouragement plagued me that day. This getting better stuff was not easy.

I was released again, after only one night, and from then on it was routine trips to the hospital to include perhaps a bag of potassium or magnesium. Then we had some issues with white cells rising too quickly and that was resolved. Actually I was doing well. Our family visited, various friends visited, and our Pastor visited. Everyone enjoyed the view, except Pastor Steve. He chose to sit back from the window while others rushed toward the windows to enjoy the sights of the city. Our grandsons would lie in the window sill inches off the floor and watch the action on the streets. Michael learned where the nearest grocery store was, and he took good care of us preparing meals. Often people would bring food prepared and ready to eat and Michael was appreciative. Cooking is not his strong point. If we finished soon enough at IPOP we would go for a ride through the neighborhoods of Baltimore. On my first ride once we were in the apartment I was craving a McDonald's cheeseburger. I have no idea why a McDonald's cheeseburger sounded so good. Michael found a McDonald's and we ate in the car. Being in a public place was not an option. Our favorite place to order food was from Pickles Pub right below our apartment building. The fried pickles are the best and Michael would head down there when company arrived. Our daily trips to IPOP were requiring less and less treatments.

One day Andy called, and said she was coming to drop something off and would not come in because she had a cold. She drove to Baltimore, parked and came to our door. She presented us with a beautiful handmade quilt made by Nancy Sauslein and her. On one side interwoven with the quilts design was various pictures of our family, and on the other side was colorful Christmas designs interwoven with Bible verses. What a precious gift, made with love that will bring years of good memories.

We began to have a day off here and there. On my birthday in December, Cindy and Steve were coming down to celebrate when we were hit by a crazy snowstorm and I-95 became an ice rink. They were forced to turn around, but we still celebrated a few days late. They are friends we can always count on. One weekend Cindy gave Michael a much needed break from his 24/7 routine and came to Baltimore to stay with me transporting me back and forth to Hopkins. Friends are definitely life's special treasures.

Christmas was coming and I was ready. Dr. Smith had told me not to plan on enjoying Thanksgiving or Christmas this year long before I entered the hospital. I had already proved him wrong and had a great Thanksgiving with my family. Now for Christmas I had done all the shopping and wrapping for everyone well in advance. Jared brought the wrapped gifts to the apartment and we celebrated together as a family.

Aiden and I even made our traditional Christmas punch. Everyone was there for Christmas Eve, and Darrell, Alisha and the boys spent the night and Christmas morning with us. Aiden had asked to sleep with me and how could I refuse. Michael and I had a king size bed in the apartment so there was plenty of room. At least I thought there was until I remembered how much a little boy can squirm in the night. I was so thankful for another Christmas with my family. I do not know why and cannot explain it, but God had been good and I was blessed.

December 30th, Day 55 was to be my last day in IPOP. Another bone marrow biopsy was done and instructions for going home were given. Michael had given January 1st as our last day in the apartment. On New Year's Eve, only because I took a long nap during the day, we stayed up and had a front row view of the Inner Harbor fireworks. It was our own private celebration there on the fifteenth floor of the Zenith of the mercy of God. Tomorrow we would go home after 65 days away.

Our sons came to help us and up the road we came. Again, I was apprehensive because of the distance from the hospital. My leash from Hopkins was lengthening. Julie and her Mom had been to our house and cleaned it from top to bottom. People had brought food and I could actually sleep in my own bed. The feelings of joy and thanksgiving were overwhelming. I was home.

We needed to return to Hopkins the next week to have my Hickman removed. That was easy and that same young doctor greeted me. My life was still very restricted. For now there was no mingling with the public, and if I stepped outside of my house, I had to wear a mask. I had purchased a wig and wore it on occasion, but actually preferred bald and so did my grandsons. So bald it was!

On one of our trips back to Hopkins, as the time between visits was rather short, we saw Ann's mom, Gretchen, in the hall. She had just stepped out of Ann's room for a moment and until that moment we did not know Ann was back in the hospital. Ann, too, had left the hospital and was able to go home and spend some time with her husband and sons while making some progress. Ann made cookies with her sons, the neighbors caroled for them. She loved her time at home and the boys and Jon loved it, too. She needed to return to Hopkins the Monday before Christmas for some more chemo and was hoping to be home again on Christmas Day. Suddenly, Ann had gotten an infection in her central nervous system. As previously stated an infection can be life threatening. Chemo had to be stopped to treat the infection and things again appeared to be going well. She got worse on Christmas Day and the next few weeks were a struggle for them all. By the end of two weeks, right before they could re-start the chemo, it became clear that the cancer without the chemo for that brief amount of time had done too much damage. Ann wasn't strong enough to do any more chemo. On January 5th the decision was made to stop treatment. The date we were at Hopkins for an appointment was January 11th. As Gretchen approached us that day we knew from her countenance the news was not good. Ann was dying. One of her final statements to her doctor had been that she hoped her doctor had learned and would continue to learn from her case anything that would help others in their fight. Ann had multiple myeloma and lost her gallant fight on January 11, 2011. Ann had impacted my life during a very brief time, but her life had reached and touched many. Ann was an architect whose projects were vast and known. She loved people and people loved her. She has two sons who will grow up knowing they had a Mom who loved them, their Dad and so many others. Jon and the boys are comforted knowing how many lives Ann touched. Ann lived her life to the fullest and was gone much too soon. Her story has forever mingled with mine. I often struggled with why Ann and not me. Once again in life those questions are God's to answer. We must trust His heart though we do not understand.

I continued to make progress in the right direction. By Day 60 the blood counts were good and the biopsy showed no cancer cells. My new marrow was working! Day 69 now settled back at home, I was officially turned back over to Dr. Hosford, but Hopkins would not cut the ties that required checking in with them on a regular basis. I could go out on limited trips still wearing the mask. I must have been a scary sight to some. By April...one year since diagnosis...I was able to be out without the mask. Sunlight and dirt were my big restrictions for fear of GVHD, bacterial, or fungal infections.

Life had changed. My blood type changed to be that of my sister. I was now considered a chimera…a Greek mythological fire -breathing she-monster composed of three animals. No, I have not turned into a fire-breathing monster, even though that could be fun at times, but my tissues do now have a different genetic constitution. The reason they use the word Chimerism (pronounced "ki") is because I now have two DNA's…my sister's bone marrow and my own cells now exist compatibly. Chimerism is the state after an allogeneic bone marrow transplant in which bone marrow (from Lynn) and my cells co-exist as the new marrow and DNA build a brand new immune system in my body. Draw blood from me and it will be my sister's DNA, scrape cells from inside my mouth and it will be my DNA. The doctor said to take life slow and adjust to the new me. At the eighteen month mark and the two year mark I would fulfill all my childhood immunizations again. I also have fought sinus infections, bronchitis, pneumonia and asthma as my new immune system grows, but there were minor compared to where I had been. I was alive and getting stronger all the time.

Today I am thankful for the cancer that tried to destroy me, but instead brought a greater appreciation for life with my family and friends. In the book of Genesis, Joseph's life was anything but easy. Yet as he revealed himself to the same brothers that had sold him into slavery so many years before, he was able to say, "…You meant evil against me, but God meant it for good…" (Genesis 50:20 NKJV) God's mercy, love, and grace still reign. Life is worth the fight!

Chapter 9

JOURNEY SINCE TRANSPLANT

My family had been consistent as my encouragers and once I was well enough to go away for a few days, I wanted us to go as a family in celebration of life. While in the hospital, I had talked of a family trip one day. Dreaming and planning for the future was important. In October, just short of a year since transplant, we planned that family trip to Washington, DC. Michael and I found a townhouse to rent close to a metro station and the plan was put into action. Everyone had some places they wanted to visit so when we all arrived on Friday afternoon; we spent the time planning our next three days touring our Capital. We had planned meals in advance with us ladies each taking a night. Saturday morning we walked to the metro and began our adventure. It did not take long for us to learn enough about the city to feel comfortable. The Capitol building, the Mall, museums, the Old Post Office, war memorials, and the Lincoln Monument to just name a few places. Aiden was extremely excited about seeing President Lincoln. The massive likeness is something everyone should see as a kid. It is a long walk to the site and Aiden carried a penny with him the entire walk so he would know for sure we had reached the right destination. We also had to see Ford's Theatre and the house where Lincoln was taken after being shot across the street and evidently died. Aiden was interested in it all. Another of his favorites was the bell tower at the Old Post Office. Eli was in the stroller, walking, or riding on someone's shoulders. He took in all the sights and sounds of the city. This was cherished time.

We saved our visit to Arlington National Cemetery for Monday. This was an emotional day for us all, especially Darrell and Jared who had experienced the trauma of war. Jared had recently lost a friend in Afghanistan and he was able to locate his grave to pay his respects. As we all walked through Arlington, the reality of war once again flooded our minds. We all had a very quiet time of reflection that day. Later we rode the metro one more time to go to eat and then said our goodbyes as Darrell, Alisha, Aiden and Eli headed back to North Carolina. Michael, Jared, Julie and I headed north for home. We all enjoyed the days together and my body had managed the walking. I was exhilarated by the accomplishments. This family trip had been a dream that became reality for me and I was once again thankful.

Becoming as strong as I can possibility be is one of my goals. I had received some information from the Leukemia and Lymphoma Society (LLS) and went to their website. As I read their information and saw how much money had been raised over the years for cancer research, I began to think perhaps this was a way I could begin to give back. Johns Hopkins is one of the many facilities that has benefited from LLS. Pouring over their information I learned of the fundraising segment called Team In Training (TNT). The idea is to take individuals on all levels and prepare them for an event while the individual raises money for LLS.

One day I had the nerve to make that first phone call. From there I was directed to the closest chapter in Bel Air, Maryland and decided to go to an informational meeting. Of course, Michael had to go with me and the event that interested me was cycling. TNT provides a coach, mentor and training schedule with the choice of several events in which to participate. That night we met Nicole and Coach Bob. I told them I was a novice cyclist with only a trail bike, but I had a willing heart. From then on I was a part of the Harford County TNT cycle team. We were a large team of ONE with Coach Bob and Mentor Nick. Knowing very little about road riding or group riding, Bob set out to teach me and I was a willing student. In February I decided to begin to train for the Fletcher Flyer in Fletcher, North Carolina. I would ride 50 miles and raise a minimum of $2,000 for LLS. Most notably I decided from the beginning I would ride in memory of Ann. Now the adventures of training with Coach Bob are vast. The next thing Michael knew I was buying a new Trek LS and moving into the big stuff. Since I was training for the Fletcher Flyer, the name Fletcher seemed appropriate for my new bike. A few minor spills and many, many miles later, I was ready to give 50 miles a shot. Coach Bob could not go to North Carolina, so my mentor, Nick, said he would go. Michael and I made the trip and enjoying every minute of the weekend. Cindy and Steve joined us and were there to cheer me on in the ride just like through the transplant. The highlight of the weekend was Gretchen, who made the trip from Raleigh, North Carolina, as I was riding for my friend, Ann, who had lost her battle. With Ann pinned to my jersey, off we went with several hundred other riders. Nick was a great riding companion encouraging me all the way. Such a sense of accomplishment as I crossed the finish line with hands held high. Gretchen placed my medal around my neck. I did it for Ann, but I did it for me, also. I was able to raise over $5,000 for LLS. One year and a half after transplant and my body cooperated.

By now, I was hooked on cycling. I continued to ride…sometimes on the trails with Will…sometimes on the road with Fletcher. So the challenge was offered to ride again in October in the Seagull Century. I signed up for the metric century. After all, I had done 50 miles on some rolling hills so I could do 62 miles on flat land. Now our team had grown from one to four. So we trained and planned and rode for weeks preparing for the trip. In October, Michael and I headed to Salisbury for the weekend and another great time. Event weekends with TNT are such a time of celebration. This time Ryan and Susan would ride with me for the duration. Once again Ann was pinned to my jersey. I never figured out how you can ride into a head wind both directions, but we did. Race completed and body exhausted, I had raised over $7,000 this year for TNT. To have my sons tell me how proud they are of me completed my experiences. There are so many amazing people I met through cycling and TNT that without having had cancer, our paths would have never crossed.

Darrell, Alisha and the boys were still living in North Carolina and Darrell was still on the 82nd Airborne Freefall Parachute jump team. In July, between cycling events, Michael and I went down to North Carolina and we both did a tandem jump with our son. Darrell and I took off in an airplane loaded with military. After they all jumped, we moved to the open door of the airplane and when the right moment came, we fell forward out of the plane. What an amazing ride to the ground from 13,500 feet with my son. We were traveling at a speed of 120 MPH after leaving the plane. Then Darrell opened the chute after a few minutes of freefall and suddenly we were in the quietest place in the universe. Darrell and I talked and he pointed out landmarks on our way to the ground. Landing was like sitting on the couch. What a wonderful experience with my son. I would do it again, too. People say why would you do such a thing after just surviving cancer? My answer is …because I am alive!

Currently, this part of my journey has brought me together with many others with a story to tell. Union Hospital now has a monthly support group meeting where I have met several new friends. As survivors and caregivers we do not waste time wallowing in our troubles knowing we always know we have each other to lean on, but we focus on the life we have been given and enjoy each other. Another group of people I would not have met without cancer. Today I, also, volunteer in the Cancer Resource Center at Union Hospital and in conjunction with the American Cancer Society to help those with cancer find the resources they require. So many great people have crossed my path, and although we too often have the sorrow of losing some to the battle, I know my life is enriched because of knowing these new friends. The losses remind us all of our humanity and the reason we strive for a cure.

Cycling continues to be a part of my life. Trail rides on "Will" or road rides on "Fletcher" are weekly events. Our Julie's brother, Jim, is an avid cyclist and we have joined up for a couple of rides, although he is so much faster. He married a sweet young lady named Alicia in 2012, and now has convinced her to ride also. As time goes on, I want to continue to ride my bikes and ride with others when possible.

Obviously, I am doing well. Since transplant my body has built a new immune system from the gift of marrow from my sister. As with anyone just two years old, viruses come easily. For this reason going back to school to teach or as a substitute is not a good idea. Although I am able to ride my bike, my stamina can be fragile. Before transplant, I had been taking some exercise classes. All the stretching, plus cardio training, had helped me to be in shape. After transplant, I slowly began those classes again. Thanks to continued cycling and exercise, my body's limits are being stretched. Setbacks come in the form of bronchitis, pneumonia, or other illness and I often find myself sick every six weeks. Perhaps licking door knobs is a way to build my immunities more quickly. There is no reason to complain because in 2010 my life was given a deadline. That deadline has come and gone and I continue to fight. My motto has been "Life is Worth the Fight" and as long as God gives me breath, I will fight.

A song, "Good to be Alive", by Jason Gray, sums up my feeling for living this life today and I want my life to demonstrate a thankful heart.

People are important to me and my family is at the top of that list. Darrell, Alisha, Aiden and Eli now live in San Antonio, Texas. Darrell is attending Physician's Assistant School and Alisha continues to support him through the long hours of school. Her job is not easy with two little ones, yet her commitment remains strong. Aiden is finished Kindergarten, playing his first year of baseball winning a first place trophy, and growing into a fine young man. Eli continues to grow and entertain us all. Even though he may be small, he is mighty and his spirit is alive. We have been able to take some trips to San Antonio and spend time with them all. Playing with the grandsons is one of my greatest joys. Aiden thinks Texas is the best place ever and tells us there is so much to do in Texas. Watching Aiden play baseball has been a special treat as well as buying the boys their first bicycles. San Antonio has some beautiful sights as we enjoyed the River Walk, The Alamo, the culture, the rodeo and the food. After Darrell completes the classroom segment, he will be moving his family again for his practicum/clinicals. At this point he will receive his commission as an officer in the Army. Our hope is for a move back to Fort Bragg. Jared and Julie continue to live in

Homeville, PA as Jared builds helicopters and Julie works for the Cecil County Soil Conservation Department helping county farmers. Jared and Julie are waiting the birth of their first child, our granddaughter, and Julie plans to quit work and be a stay-at-home Mom for now. I, too, am anxiously waiting. Michael and I continue to enjoy this life we have been given.

Jared and Julie wanted to tell us all in a unique way the sex of the baby. Julie baked a cake, filled it with a special filling, and decorated it beautifully as it was covered in pink and blue question marks. Her family and Grandmom Owens gathered at her parent's house for the revealing. Michael and I were at Darrell and Alisha's house in Texas so we set a time for the cake cutting and joined them all on Skype. Julie cut the cake to everyone's squeals that it is a girl. She had filled the cake with pink filling. We were all excited to be a part of the announcement. Eighty Eight year old, Grandmom Owens announced, "I have never been invited to a sex party before!" Once again good memories were made with the family and technology played an important part.

Spring and summer bring more time with family and friends. Michael and I celebrate our 40th wedding anniversary on June 9th, 2013. Alisha and the boys come to Maryland to spend a month after Aiden graduates from kindergarten. We share the time with Alisha's family as we all have some fun days with Aiden, Eli and Alisha. We love our grandchildren, but enjoy equally our time with Darrell, Alisha, Jared and Julie. Michael celebrated his 65th birthday on June 25th. I actually surprised him with a party. Several family members and friends attended the party. Watching my family play and interact with each other always makes me smile.

Another important day occurred with the shower for Julie and Jared. Several people were involved in the giving of the shower and it was a fantastic day with family and friends as Liza will be well clothed for her first year, along with many practical gifts for Liza's Mommy and Daddy. Grandmom Owens, through her church, allowed us to use the community house for the shower. During the preparations on the day of the shower, Grandmom told us that 65 years ago she had been given a shower in that same building also in the month of June as she awaited the birth of her son and Liza's Granddaddy, Michael. Circles continue.

July allowed us to spend some time with my parents, sisters, and family in Wisconsin as my sister, Lynn, who was able to fly in from Denver. It was time with my family that was well-spent and needed. Before we left for the trip, Julie was having some contractions. I simply asked Liza to please wait until we returned from Wisconsin as I have blocked out the entire month of August for her. Liza complied...so we wait.

THE BIRTH OF FIRST GRANDDAUGHTER

The birth of our granddaughter, Liza Jane Owens, seems to be the place to wrap up this book. New life always means life continues on. God's grace and mercy shine through a newborn baby's cry. Birth is a miracle.

On Monday, August 12th, and after Julie's ultrasound, Jared called to say they were being admitted to labor and delivery at the hospital. Soon we were on our way to Jennersville, PA to see what exactly was happening. The hospital is only about a twenty minute ride from our house. We found Julie attached to monitors and receiving fluids as decisions were being made on how to proceed. Contractions were beginning. Julie's Mom, Janice, Michael and I joined Jared and Julie in the wait. Later in the evening, Janice, Michael and I were told we should go home and get some sleep as this could be a long twenty four to thirty six hours. Meanwhile Julie's Dad, David, went to their house to pick up their dog, Penny, so she would be cared for over the next few days. The birth seemed to still be many hours away as we left them to go home. We Moms promised to have our cell phones close and were promised a call if anything changed.

At 4:00 a.m. our phone rang. It was Jared telling us that things were progressing and we should make our way to the hospital. He also had called Janice and David. Michael and I got ready, grabbed an oatmeal bar and headed north, with the plan to stop for coffee on the way. It was storming and often raining quite hard. Perhaps it was those trumpets blowing at the birth of another grandchild. At 4:39 a.m., I received a text saying, "happening soon, I think". So much for the coffee as we by- passed Wawa heading for Jennersville arriving before 5:00 a.m. We had to wait for security to take us up upstairs and as we finally reached the floor, Jared came around the curtain to ask if we had seen Janice. Now I was beginning to panic. We all lived so close and this was to be Janice and David's first grandchild. I certainly did not want them to miss this event! Finally Janice and David arrived with great sighs of relief from us all. We were all there! Janice and I took our places in the room with Jared and Julie as David and Michael stood in the hallway listening intently to everything. During the birth there was actually a severe weather warning broadcast that came in on three of our phones. That was the first time any of us received these warnings and Julie was not happy with the alarms sounding from our otherwise silenced cellphones. At 5:25 a.m., on August 13, 2013, Julie gave birth to Liza Jane Owens weighing 5 pounds, 15 ounces and 20 inches long. Liza's first cry was heard by all, as an emotional Dad and grandparents watched and listened. Michael said David had tears running down his cheeks as the emotions of the moment took control. Julie did amazingly well and Liza came much faster than anyone had predicted. Jared was able to cut the cord and Liza was placed on her Mommy's chest. This was another incredible experience to have the honor of being present at the birth of our third grandchild and first granddaughter!

Liza Jane Owens, as I reflect on the miracle of your birth and the love your family has for you, the following verse comes to mind. **Psalms 103:8 ESV "The Lord is merciful and gracious, slow to anger and abounding in steadfast love."** Just as you will grow to know your family's unchangeable love for you, may you learn to understand God's abounding love!

Perhaps more grandchildren will come later for both our sons and their families, and each one will be welcomed and loved. I am blessed to be called Nana, married to Granddaddy and for the privilege of still being here to know Aiden, Eli, and Liza.

Remember those twist and turns of the churning storm referred to earlier? We do not know the future, but remain firm in our belief that

God is in control. Life continues to bring us the unexpected. Michael and I travel this journey together, though valleys lie ahead, as he now faces cancer. In the midst of trouble always lies a blessing. None of us know what is around the next turn. We, together, have much to learn. We want our lives to reflect our confidence is in God alone.

Psalms 61:2-3 NKJV "…when my heart is overwhelmed; lead me to the rock that is higher than I. For You have been a shelter for me…"

My insecurities can still be present and people pleasing can still get me into trouble. Acknowledging God each day helps to maintain my focus. This journey was never guaranteed to be easy. God has proven faithful, yet often I still waiver in my trust of Him. My desire is to continue to grow mentally and spiritually, and to stay physically active. Grumpy old people are a sad sight, and I want to live out my days smiling and content with whatever may come my way and, if possible, leave this world satisfied and saying "It has been a great journey".

Psalms 16:11 NKJV "You will show me the path of life; in your presence is fullness of joy; at your right hand are pleasures forevermore."

Chapter 10

JOURNEY YET UNSEEN

Hebrews 11:1 KJV "Now faith is the substance of things hoped for, the evidence of things not seen."

Without the knowledge of God and His Son, Jesus Christ, my life would be without meaning and the storm would be too much. This knowledge was essential as I have traveled this journey. I rest in the assurance that one day I will be with Him and all those unanswered questions will either be answered or unimportant. My faith rests on the foundation that began long before the world's existence and the assurance that God always keep His promises. Nothing; struggles, war, cancer or death can separate me from the love of God. (Read Romans 8:38-39)

Recently, as I was taking a walk with my grandsons, Aiden and Eli, we talked about many different things as usual. We discussed why the sky is blue, where all these pretty rocks came from and how many steps is it from our house to the neighbors. You never know what statements or questions will come from these little guys and they continually make life interesting. Six year old Aiden, only a couple of weeks earlier, after a conversation with his Mom and Dad, had asked Jesus to come live in his heart as he is tender toward the things of God. On this day a few weeks later, he began asking me questions about heaven. The following is our conversation.

"Nana, I asked Jesus to come live in my heart. You know He died for me, right?"

"Yes, I do, Aiden. I am so glad to know that!"

"Nana, what are we going to do in heaven?'

I replied, "I am not sure, but I know it will be a great place because Jesus is preparing it for us now."

"Nana, a girl at school said her grandmother just died."

"I'm sorry to hear that, Aiden."

"Nana, will you go to heaven when you die?"

"Sure will, Aiden, because Jesus made the way to heaven plain and simple, and I asked Him to be in my life. I will be waiting for you when I get there."

Really,' He replied excitedly. "So when you die I will get to see you again?" Watching him light up at the realization of being together again someday was very special.

"Yes, you will. Someday we will all be together again."

My salvation is sure and my eternal life is secure not based on anything I have done, but on the ultimate sacrifice of God's only begotten Son for my sins and the sins of the entire world. That day on the porch with Mom, though I was only a child, my eternal journey began and this journey has no end. Heaven is beyond our imagination and one day I plan to spend it with all of you.

John 3:16-17 NKJV

"For God so loved the world that he gave his only begotten son, that whosoever believes in him should not perish but have everlasting life."

"For God did not send His Son into the world to condemn the world, but that the world through Him might be saved."

Psalms 17:15 NKJV

"As for me, I will see your face in righteousness; I shall be satisfied when I awake in your likeness."

Revelation 5:13b NKJV

"…Blessing and honor, and glory and power be to him that sits on the throne and to the Lamb forever and ever."

Epilogue

Read and reread Proverbs Chapter Three. There are so many nuggets of truth secured in this one chapter for our daily lives. Obeying, remembering, trusting, honoring and being wise in God's eyes and not our own, are found in this one chapter. Learning to live out God's truths daily remains our goal as the storm continues.

To be continued...

I still have goals and dreams to fulfill:

...Growing old with Michael as he and I face physical battles together.

...Demonstrating the Grace of God to others around me.

...Enjoying times with my sons and daughters-in-law that God has given us.

...Watching my grandsons grow to young men and seeing my granddaughter grow to a young lady and perhaps have more grandchildren!

...Playing more games with my family.

...Spending more time with the friends I am blessed to know.

...Flying in a helicopter with Jared.

...Cycling many miles on my road bike and trail bike.

...Taking more trips with Michael to places we have yet to see.

...Giving more time to others.

...Living this life with a thankful heart for all I have been given.

...Creating more memories!

...Leaving this world smiling and content!

All the credit for this journey belongs to God.

Consider the following websites and suggestions to see what you can do to help others:

LEUKEMIA AND LYMPHOMA SOCIETY
Team in Training

THE NATIONAL BONE MARROW REGISTRY
Be the Match.com

AMERICAN CANCER SOCIETY
ACS.com

BE AN ORGAN DONOR

ALSO CONSIDER VOLUNTEERING... YOUR CHURCH AND YOUR COMMUNITY IS ALWAYS LOOKING FOR COMMITTED VOLUNTEERS.

Family Pictures

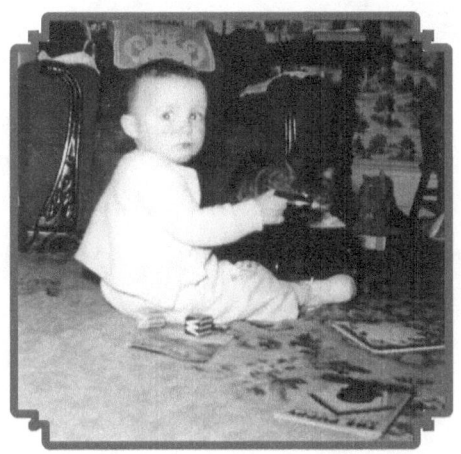

Donna – December 1953
Criswell farm

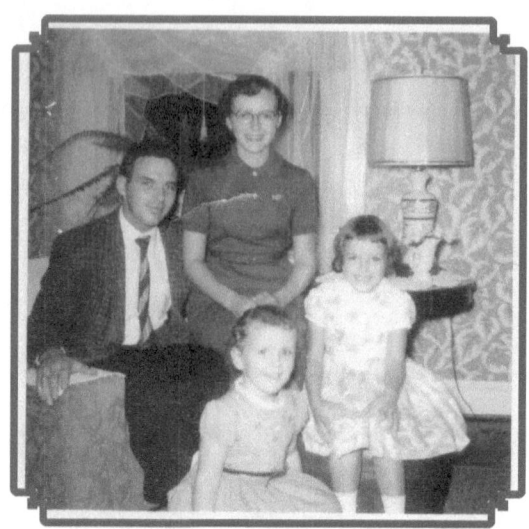

Dad, Mom, Lynn and Donna 1958
Lynn would one day become my marrow donor as a perfect match.

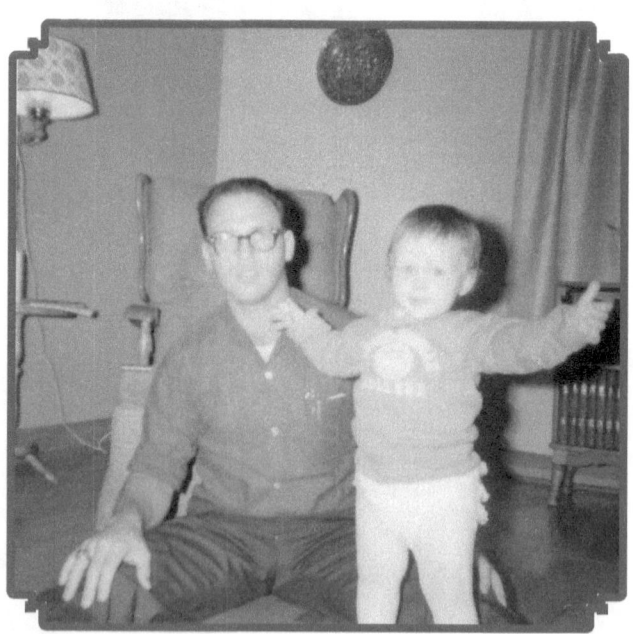

Dad and Deneen – 1965 in Tennessee

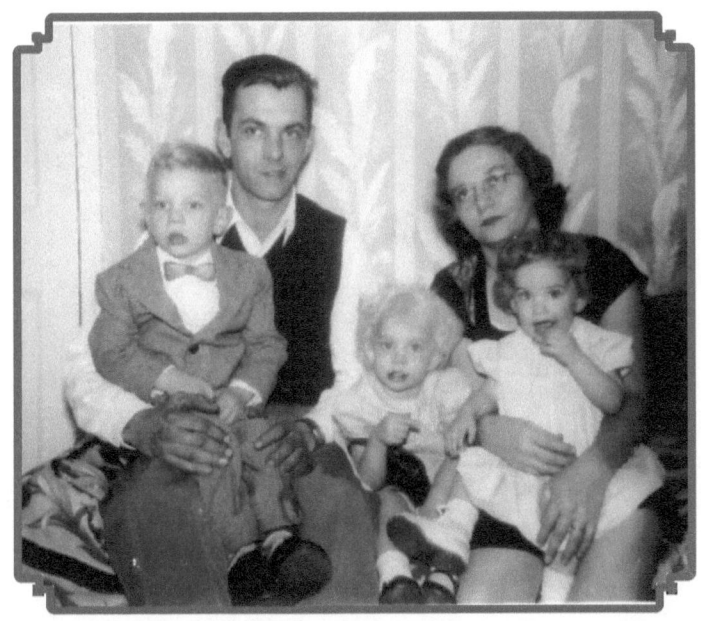

Michael, his Dad, Alfred, Sharon, his Mom, Kathleen, and Charlotte 1954

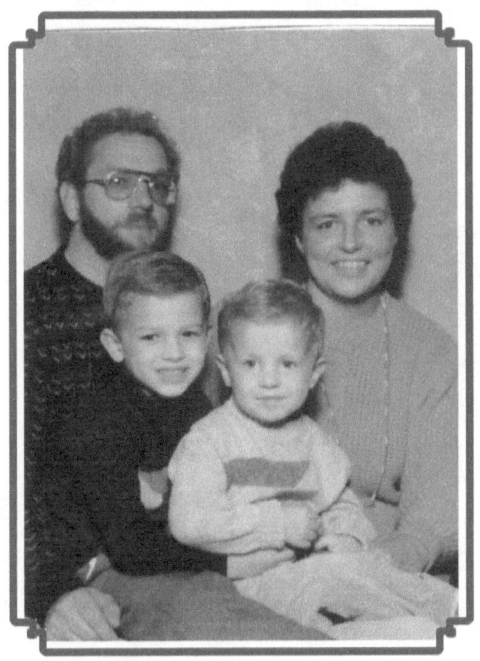

Michael, Donna, Darrell and Jared 1986

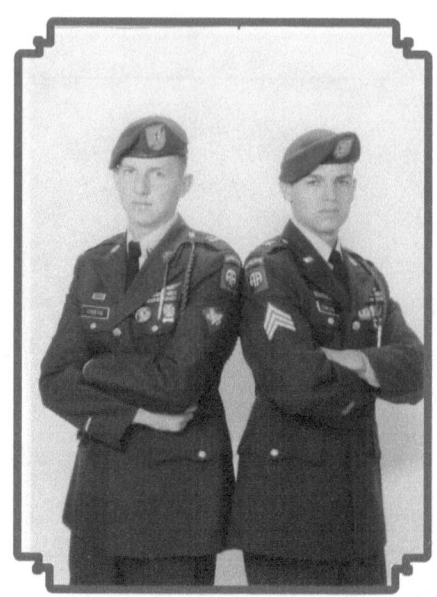

Jared and Darrell
United States Army
82nd Airborne Division, Fort Bragg, North Carolina
2003

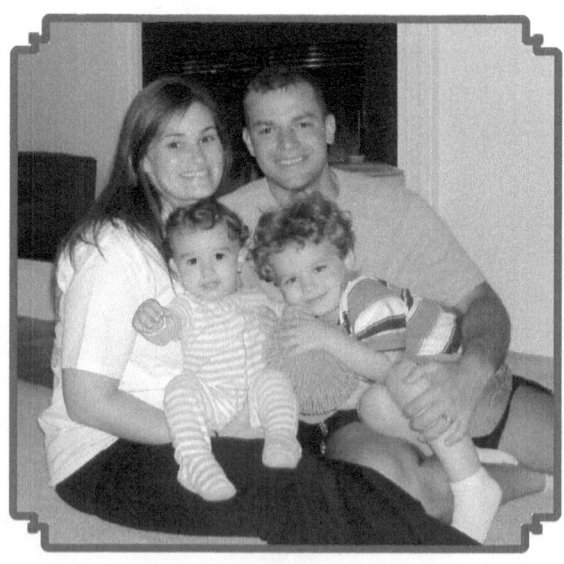

Alisha, Darrell, Eli and Aiden
Sanford, North Carolina May 2011

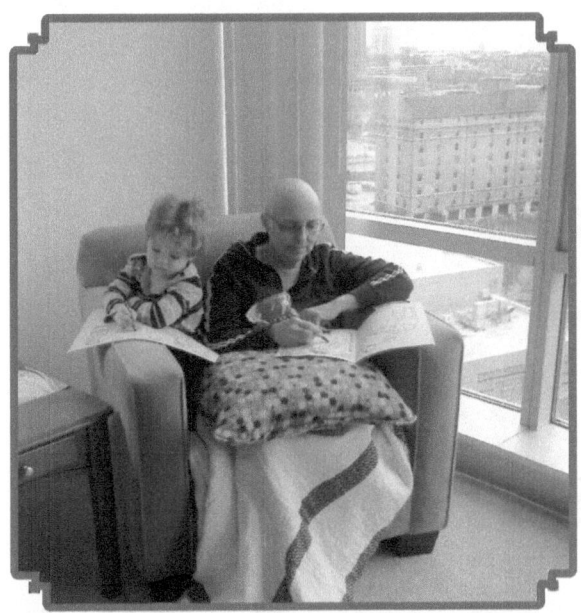

Donna recovering from bone marrow transplant
Aiden and Donna coloring – November 2010
Zenith Apartments – Pratt Street, Baltimore, MD
The warehouse at Camden Yards is in the background.

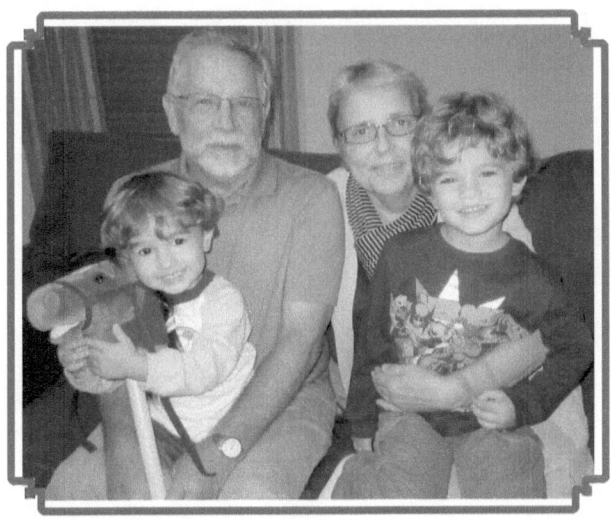

Granddaddy, Nana and Grandsons, Aiden and Eli
San Antonio, TX October, 2012

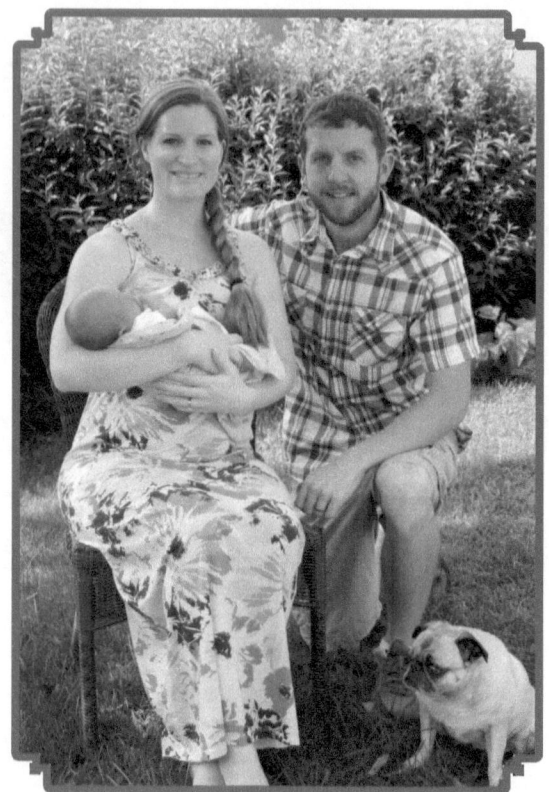

Julie, Liza, Jared and their dog, Penny
August 20, 2013

Bibliography

Cowman, L.B. Streams in the Desert, Zondervan Corporation, 1996.

Famous Quotes and Authors.com/copyright 2011/Benjamin Franklin Quote

Guys and Dolls; musical by Frank Loesser/ "A Bushel and A Peck", Published in 1950.